MYplace

Published by First Place for Health
Galveston, Texas, USA
www.firstplaceforhealth.com
Printed in the USA

ISBN: 978-1-942425-52-6

CONTENTS

MY PLACE FOR BIBLE STUDY
Fit for a King

FOREWORD

I was introduced to First Place for Health in 1993 by my mother-in-law, who had great concern for the welfare of her grandchildren. I was overweight and overwrought! God used that first Bible study to start me on my journey to health, wellness, and a life of balance.

Our desire at First Place for Health is for you to begin that same journey. We want you to experience the freedom that comes from an intimate relationship with Jesus Christ and witness His love for you through reading your Bible and through prayer. To this end, we have designed each day's study (which will take about fifteen to twenty minutes to complete) to help you discover the deep truths of the Bible. Also included is a weekly Bible memory verse to help you hide God's Word in your heart. As you start focusing on these truths, God will begin a great work in you.

At the beginning of Jesus' ministry, when He was teaching from the book of Isaiah, He said to the people, "The Spirit of the Lord is on me, because he has anointed me to preach good news to the poor. He has sent me to proclaim freedom for the prisoners and recovery of sight for the blind, to release the oppressed, to proclaim the year of the Lord's favor" (Luke 4:18–19). Jesus came to set us free—whether that is from the chains of compulsivity, addiction, gluttony, overeating, under eating, or just plain unbelief. It is our prayer that He will bring freedom to your heart so you may experience abundant life.

God bless you as you begin this journey toward a life of liberty.

Vicki Heath, First Place for Health National Director

ABOUT THE AUTHOR

Debbie Behling joined First Place (the original name for First Place for Health) at Houston's First Baptist Church in 1981, the year it began. She became a leader the following year, and she started groups in two other locations. Currently she leads a group at Sugar Land Methodist Church in Texas, which has been meeting since 2005.

Debbie taught middle school social studies for 19 years and high school social studies online for 11 years. For 16 years she worked as an education specialist with Region 4 Education Service Center, creating numerous professional development sessions and presenting at local, state, national, and international conferences. She authored, co-authored, and/or edited over 30 publications for Region 4 between 2003 and 2018. Since then she has authored *The Joy Adventure*, *God My Refuge*, and *A Better Way* Bible studies for First Place for Health.

Debbie earned a B.A. from Dallas Baptist College in 1977 with a triple major in secondary education, history, and psychology. Her postgraduate degree is an M.Ed. with a focus on educational technology from Northwestern University in Natchitoches, Louisiana.

In 2018 she retired from full-time employment after 35 years in education. She lives in Sugar Land, Texas, with her husband and brood of miniature dachshunds and has two children and one grandson. She loves to lead her First Place for Health group, write, sing in the church choir, scrapbook, travel, and research genealogy. Her social media handle is @bdebsing.

ABOUT THE CONTRIBUTOR

Lisa Lewis, who provided the menus and recipes in this study, is the author of *Healthy Happy Cooking*. Lisa's cooking skills have been a part of First Place for Health wellness weeks and other events for many years. She provided recipes for seventeen of the First Place for Health Bible studies and is a contributing author in *Better Together* and *Healthy Holiday Living*. She partners with community networks, including the Real Food Project, to bring healthy cooking classes to underserved areas. She is dedicated to bringing people together around the dinner table with healthy, delicious meals that are easy to prepare. Lisa lives in Galveston and is married to John. They have three children: Tal, Hunter, and Harper. Visit www.healthyhappycook.com for more delicious inspiration.

INTRODUCTION

First Place for Health is a Christ-centered health program that emphasizes balance in the physical, mental, emotional, and spiritual areas of life. The First Place for Health program is meant to be a daily process. As we learn to keep Christ first in our lives, we will find that He is the One who satisfies our hunger and our every need.

This Bible study is designed to be used in conjunction with the First Place for Health program but can be beneficial for anyone interested in obtaining a balanced lifestyle. The Bible study has been created in a seven-day format, with the last two days reserved for reflection on the material studied. Keep in mind that the ultimate goal of studying the Bible is not only for knowledge but also for application and a changed life. Don't feel anxious if you can't seem to find the correct answer. Many times, the Word will speak differently to different people, depending on where they are in their walk with God and the season of life they are experiencing. Be prepared to discuss with your fellow First Place for Health members what you learned that week through your study.

There are some additional components included with this study that will be helpful as you pursue the goal of giving Christ first place in every area of your life:

- **Leader Discussion Guide:** This discussion guide is provided to help the First Place for Health leader guide a group through this Bible study. It includes ideas for facilitating a First Place for Health class discussion for each week of the Bible study.

- **Jump Start Recipes:** There are seven days of recipes--breakfast, lunch and dinner-- to get you started.

- **Steps for Spiritual Growth:** This section will provide you with some basic tips for how to memorize Scripture and make it a part of your life, establish a quiet time with God each day, and share your faith with others..

- **First Place for Health Member Survey:** Fill this out and bring it to your first meeting. This information will help your leader know your interests and talents.

- **Personal Weight and Measurement Record:** Use this form to keep a record of your weight loss. Record any loss or gain on the chart after the weigh-in at each week's meeting.

○ **Weekly Prayer Partner Forms:** Fill out this form before class and place it into a basket during the class meeting. After class, you will draw out a prayer request form, and this will be your prayer partner for the week. Try to call or email the person sometime before the next class meeting to encourage that person.

○ **100-Mile Club:** A worthy goal we encourage is for you to complete 100 miles of exercise during your nine weeks in First Place for Health. There are many activities listed that count toward your goal of 100 miles and a handy tracker to track your miles.

○ **Live It Trackers:** Your Live It Tracker is to be completed at home and turned in to your leader at your weekly First Place for Health meeting. The Tracker is designed to help you practice mindfulness and stay accountable with regard to your eating and exercise habits.

WEEK ONE: DAVID'S CALLING

SCRIPTURE MEMORY VERSE

God testified concerning him: "I have found David son of Jesse, a man after my own heart; he will do everything I want him to do." Acts 13:22

If you could be like anyone in the Bible, other than Jesus, who would it be? I have two personal favorites. Joseph is first, because he was faithful to God through many horrendous trials, delivered from prison, exalted to leadership, and finally reunited with his family. Those are qualities and outcomes I'd like to realize. The other person I'd like to emulate is Daniel. He was consistently faithful to God in a foreign land, dedicated in prayer, and delivered from the lion's den and never compromised his commitment to God. Perhaps Job exemplified characteristics you'd like to follow: faithful to God through suffering and commended by God for his humility. Or women like Deborah, Ruth, and Esther, who followed God in the midst of disasters and overcame great odds.

David would not be in my top three people after whom to pattern my life. Although there are amazing stories of David slaying a giant, writing great psalms, and serving as God's chosen king, he also committed adultery and murder. He was sometimes bold and a man of action, sometimes melancholy and passive, sometimes faithful, sometimes disobedient. He was humble but flawed. The Bible lays out his life, warts and all. More pages in the Hebrew Bible are about him than another person, and he is mentioned more than anyone in the entire Bible except Jesus. But despite David's life being a mixture of good and bad, God made him king of Israel and said that David was "a man after my own heart" (Acts 13:22). What could it mean to be a person after God's heart who conquers giants but can't conquer his own lusts? If I'm honest, I'm more like David than Joseph or Daniel. I want to become a person who is fit for serving the King, our Father God, the King of Kings, and Lord of Lords. I want to be consistently obedient, make healthy choices, and reach my fitness goals. The *Fit for a King* Bible study explores this process by examining David's life, studying his capabilities, choices, and characteristics, and making connections to our lives today. Through this investigation, we can further develop our objective of seeking God first in our lives and loving Him with our whole being. He is calling us to be a person who is fit to be a king who serves Him and His people well. Let's discover what that means and how it can empower us to make healthy choices.

—— DAY 1: GOD'S CHOICE

My gracious Father, You are the one and only great and mighty God. I'm so thankful You love me and desire to speak to me today. I bow before You, anticipating Your life-giving words of hope and strength during this quiet time with You.

He was not a good-looking man. When people saw him in person for the first time, they were shocked by his dramatic physical features: tall and lanky, misshapen nose, heavy eyebrows that drooped over his eyes. His clothes hung loosely on his tall, ungainly frame. He had an unsightly mole on his right cheek and his skin was rough and leathery. His voice was high and thin. If Abraham Lincoln ran for president today, it is unlikely he could win, because candidates today are judged harshly on the basis of their appearance. But Lincoln proved to be an effective leader during our nation's greatest crisis, the Civil War, and the country reunited under his presidency. Although his looks were lacking, his achievements were amazing.

Physical appearances can be deceiving. This is a lesson that Samuel the prophet learned during a critical time in Israel's history. Saul was a tall, handsome man who served as Israel's first king. But he turned out to be a great disappointment. Due to his rebellion against God, He chose to replace Saul and He called Samuel to anoint His new king. Turn to 1 Samuel 16. In verse 5 Samuel met Jesse and his sons and began to determine which one of them would be Israel's new leader. What does verse 6 say about Samuel's assessment of Jesse's sons?

_____

_____

_____

What is God's response in verse 7?

_____

_____

_____

God's calling doesn't always follow our preconceived notions. Although the society of the time placed greater value on the firstborn in a family, God often chose a different child for His purposes: Abel, Jacob, Joseph, Moses, and David. Samuel himself was not the firstborn of his father, yet God called him to serve as the last leader in the era of the judges of Israel.

You likely are a member of First Place for Health because you want to lose weight. Why do people want to lose weight? Initially they do because they don't like the way they look or the way their clothes fit. They are looking at the outside but God is looking on the inside, searching for a person fit for royalty. He wants to change you from the inside out. He is calling you to seek Him first in all things and love Him with all your being. Read 2 Timothy 1:9; what does it say about our calling?

_____

_____

_____

Ephesians 1:18-19 also refers to our calling. What do we learn from these verses?

_____

_____

_____

Finally find 1 Thessalonians 5:24 and identify the characteristics of the One Who calls us.

_____

_____

_____

Outwardly, David was just a shepherd boy, the youngest son in his family. But God chose and called him over all his older brothers. Just as David was called to be king of Israel, we are also called to a special place in God's kingdom. When we place our faith in Christ, we are set apart for His purposes. That is what being a "saint" or "holy" means: not perfect but providentially picked to fulfill a unique purpose, becoming more like Him every day. It does not mean the best looking, the most prominent, or the most popular. It does not mean the thinnest, the most glamourous, or the most successful. You are called by God to a royal position no matter how you look or how much you weigh. Your calling depends on God and the power Jesus imparts to you through His death and resurrection.

God knew from the beginning that David would be a man after His own heart, so He knew he was fit to be Israel's king. Write this week's memory verse here.

_____

_____

_____

People who are fit for a king are ready to answer His call to love Him with all they are. How can you answer God's call to make healthy choices today?

Thank You, Father, for your call in my life. I want to answer Your call and fulfill Your purposes for me. Help me to follow Your call today as I seek You first in all things. Amen.

—— DAY 2: A SHEPHERD'S HEART

You are my Shepherd, Lord, and I want for nothing. Thank You for leading me beside quiet waters and into Your lush green pastures. Speak to my heart now as I stop and listen to You.

God decided a shepherd boy was fit to be the king to lead His people. Shepherds were considered to be one of the lowest professions in the society of David's time. First, let's read 1 Samuel 17:34-35. What are the characteristics of a shepherd that translated into a king's role? What did David say that could connect to his ability to lead?

A shepherd's heart is *protective*: brave and willing to take risks. He will go to any lengths to keep his sheep from danger. What did Jesus say about Himself as the Good Shepherd in John 10:11-16?

Jesus also calls Himself the sheep gate in John 10:7. A shepherd would create a pen for his sheep by piling rocks around a perimeter. He would leave an opening for the sheep to go in and come out. To protect the sheep during the night, the shepherd himself would lie down in the opening so he would be ready to shield the sheep from attack. The shepherd defended his flock by literally being the door of the pen.

A second characteristic of a shepherd can be found in Psalm 23. What does the shepherd do for the sheep in this passage? Complete the blanks below. (These blanks follow the NIV; feel free to adjust them to match whatever translation you choose.)

The Lord is my _____; I _____. (verse 1)

He makes me to _____ in green _____, (verse 2)

he leads me beside _____, (verse 2)

he _____ my soul. (verse 3)

You prepare a _____ before me in the presence of my _____. (verse 5)

You _____ my head with _____; my cup _____. (verse 5)

A shepherd's heart *provides*. Sheep on their own could not survive without a place to graze and water to drink. The area where David lived was quite barren. Land that had decent rainfall was used for farming. So shepherds had to search out areas where there was grass for their sheep to eat, often walking for miles just to find a bit of pasture. Sheep are easily frightened so a calm pond rather than a flowing stream is needed for them to drink. Oil was used to soothe scrapes and heal cuts. The shepherd was always looking out for the needs of his sheep, and it was a full-time job. In the same way God provides for us: meeting our needs and giving us what we need. What does Philippians 4:19 say about this truth?

_____

_____

_____

Finally, let's finish examining Psalm 23 for a third characteristic of a shepherd. Complete the blanks below.

He guides me along the _____ for his name's sake. (verse 3)

Even though I walk through the _____, I will _____

no _____, for you are _____; your _____ and

your _____, they _____ me. (verse 4)

Surely your _____ and _____ will follow me all the days of my

_____, and I will _____ in the _____

of the Lord _____. (verse 6)

A shepherd's heart allows him to be *present*. David would have been with his sheep through every possible condition: thwarting attacks by predators, searching for food and water, and sleeping with them at night. He disciplined them with his rod and directed them with his staff. He knew his sheep well, and they knew him. What does

Jesus say about Himself as the Good Shepherd in John 10:3-5?

_____

_____

_____

Being a shepherd taught David to protect, provide for, and be present for his sheep. These characteristics would serve him well during his reign as king. We will learn more about these facets of David's character later in this study. As we end our time together today, let's meditate on how God protects, provides, and is present for us. The Good Shepherd is all we ever need to guide us on our wellness journey.

Thank You for your protection, provision, and presence, Father. I truly have everything that I need because You are my Good Shepherd. Lead me in Your paths today and empower me to put You above all others. Amen.

—— DAY 3: A MUSICIAN'S HEART
My heart sings with joy as I enter into Your presence, my God. I am eager to hear Your voice and excited about what I will learn as I meet with You.

I got into my car after a visit to my podiatrist. He had determined that I needed surgery on my foot to correct three unrelated issues. I would wear a boot for six weeks during one of the busiest times of the year at work, when I would be standing for hours to engage teachers in professional development sessions. As I started the car to drive to work, I was mulling over how I would handle this challenge. I turned on the radio and heard a song by Sandi Patti that talked about beautiful feet. I laughed out loud at the gift God gave me at that moment through music. I felt encouraged and joyful, reminded that my God was with me even through this trial.

Music impacts us in amazing ways. It activates all four parts of our being: emotional, spiritual, mental, and physical. It has the power to "promote well-being, enhance learning, stimulate cognitive function, improve quality of life, and even induce happiness."[1] God created music to connect every part of our being to Him. The encouraging effect of music is one reason I include songs in each Day 7 lesson of the Bible studies I write. Let's look at a few examples of music in the Bible. Find each scripture in the following chart and describe how music is being used.

Scripture	How Music Is Used
Exodus 15	
Mark 14:22-26 (verse 26)	
Revelation 5:8-10	

How does music impact you? What is a favorite song that connects you to God and why?

_____

_____

_____

A kingly heart, a heart like God's, is full of music, expressions of emotions that connect the four parts of our being with Him. You don't have to be a musician or be able to sing to allow God's music to impact you. Listening to music can connect you to God, and attending worship and praise gatherings connects you with your Christian family members. Plugging in your earbuds to play music while you exercise brings all the benefits of music together at once.

David was a gifted musician. He wrote lyrics and melodies, sang, and played the lyre, a stringed instrument that was held upright and strummed. God used his musical abilities to bring him into the king's inner circle and continue his calling. Read 1 Samuel 16:14-23 and describe how David became the court musician.

_____

_____

_____

We will explore more of David's music later in this study. Part of his calling was to use God's gift of music in his life for His purposes. What gift or gifts has He given you to use for His glory? How do you express your love for God in creative ways?

_____

_____

_____

Thank You for the gift of music, Father, and for the way You use it in my life to bring me closer to You. As I walk through this day, sing Your song through me and guide me as I seek You first. Amen.

DAY 4: A KING'S HEART

You are my King, Father God, strong and mighty to save. I worship You, worthy Lord, and kneel before Your awesome presence as I listen now to Your Word.

God's calling of David to become Israel's king didn't start with his meeting with the prophet Samuel. He was destined to be king from before his birth. From what Israeli tribe did David come (1 Chronicles 2:3, 13-14)?

_____

What does Genesis 49:10 say about this tribe of Israel?

_____

_____

Yet after Samuel anointed David as king, it was many years before he ascended to the throne. King Saul hunted him down many times, he fled to the Philistines' land to escape him, and he struggled against those from the other eleven tribes who wanted Saul's family to continue ruling after Saul's death. What was it about David's heart that made him fit to be God's choice as king, a great leader of His chosen people?

Read 1 Samuel 16:13; after his anointing, what did David have with him?

_____

First, the heart of the king is *led by God's Spirit*. Because we are His children, we are empowered by the Holy Spirit. Unlike David, we are blessed with a constant indwelling of the Spirit. He is always in us, ready to guide us and give us strength to carry out God's will. Look up John 14:16-17; what does Jesus say about the Holy Spirit?

_____

_____

_____

Now find 1 Samuel 17:17-20. What did David's father tell him to do?

_____

_____

_____

Second, a king's heart is *ready to serve*. Notice that after David's anointing he was still working as a shepherd in his father's household. He didn't quit his day job. David was not lording it over his brothers, knowing he was to become king. He didn't wear a T-shirt identifying himself as the anointed leader of Israel. David responded obediently to whatever task God had for him. Nothing was beneath his dignity in his service to God. He didn't see the kingship as an excuse for not taking care of small tasks when he was called to do them. How does Colossians 3:17 relate to David's attitude?

_____

_____

_____

Finally, let's look at back at 1 Samuel 16:14-23 from yesterday's lesson. David served in the king's court as his musician before his own reign as king began, before anyone other than his family knew about his anointing. A king's heart is *pure in motive*. David knew God had called him to be the next king, but he served the current king faithfully. He could have used that opportunity to further his own position but he didn't. He could have worked against the king during the times that an evil spirit tormented him but he didn't. He could have talked about the king to others to embarrass or undermine him but he didn't. David trusted God to do whatever He wanted and use him in any way He chose. He didn't feel the need to help God accomplish His plan. His submission to God made him fit for the king's throne he would occupy.

So David's life shows us that a person fit to be a king called by God is *led by His Spirit*, *ready to serve*, and *pure in motive*. These attitudes came from humble trust in God as his King rather than selfishly being his own man. We can learn from David's response to God's calling. We can choose to put God first in all things, including our food and exercise choices. He has called us all to be leaders in our spheres of influence. People who know we are following God in our health journeys look to us for encouragement and example. They see the results of our faithfulness to Him. How is God using your participation in First Place for Health to influence others to follow Him?

_____

_____

_____

Check my heart, God. How well am I being led by the Spirit, serving You faithfully, and following You with pure motives? You are calling me to live for You so others will be drawn to You. I respond to Your call in faith and humility like David. Help me to seek You first today. Amen.

—— DAY 5: GOD'S CALLING

You have called me to this quiet time today, Holy God. My heart needs Your calming touch as I separate myself from the world to be still before You. I'm ready to hear what You have to say to me.

Read Psalm 78:70-72. How does Asaph, the writer of this psalm, summarize David's calling?

_____

_____

_____

Imagine David out in the fields tending his sheep. It started as an ordinary day. He was involved in his normal routine. Suddenly someone came to take his place as he was called to the house. He was surprised to find that Samuel, the great prophet of Israel, was there and wanted to see him. Samuel poured oil over his head and told him he would become the next king of Israel. Then Samuel left with no further directions to this future leader. What do you think went through David's mind and heart?

_____

_____

_____

Did David wonder what he should do next? There was no orientation manual for future kings of Israel. The current king was not a good role model for him and didn't yet know he was going to be replaced by David. Was he afraid or anxious? We don't know the answers to these questions, but we do know that God called him right then and there. The New Testament writers give us insight about being called by God and our response to that calling. Look up the scriptures on the chart and record what each says about God's calling for Christians.

Scripture	God's Calling for Christians
Romans 11:29	
Ephesians 4:1-2	
1 Peter 1:13-15	

The bar is pretty high: be holy like God. How is that possible? Even David didn't remain sinless throughout his entire life after his calling. God does not call us without providing us with what we need to fulfill His call. Hundreds of years later, in the same town where David lived, Jesus was born. What was Jesus's calling? Read 1 John 4:14 to find the answer.

_____

_____

_____

Our calling to be holy like Jesus comes with the power of the Holy Spirit living in us. We can consistently make healthy choices because of His resurrection power, an amazing result of Jesus' obedience to His calling. His sacrifice created a new bond between God and His creation. Look up John 1:12-13; what is our relationship with God through Jesus?

_____

_____

_____

Reverend John Schultz makes this connection between David and Jesus.

As a young Christian, living in the Netherlands, I met an American preacher who paid a good deal of attention to me and showed me unusual affection. I found out that I reminded him of his son, who was the same age I was, whom he had left behind in the United States and, evidently, missed during his overseas trip. We could say that David reminded God of His own Son, Jesus Christ, and that this was the main reason why He paid so much attention to this shepherd boy.[2]

God called David from the shepherd's field to the king's throne, and He was with him every step of the way. We can be confident of the same thing: God has called us and will walk with us every moment as we seek Him first. 2 Timothy 1:9-10 says,

> [God] has saved us and called us to a holy life—not because of anything we have done but because of his own purpose and grace. This grace was given us in Christ Jesus before the beginning of time, but it has now been revealed through the appearing of our Savior, Christ Jesus, who has destroyed death and has brought life and immortality to light through the gospel.

May we walk daily in our calling as God's children as the Spirit leads and empowers us to live holy lives and make healthy choices.

I am overwhelmed that You have called me to be Your child, dear Father. And I want to respond well to that calling, living in a way that reflects Your glory and Your holiness. Walk with me today as I depend on Your Holy Spirit in my fitness and faith journey, keeping my eyes always on You. Amen.

—— DAY 6: REFLECTION AND APPLICATION
Oh God, You are my God, and I earnestly seek You. I want to learn to walk in Your ways daily and not my own. Speak to me now and give me all I need to follow You.

Practice reciting this week's memory verse here.

_____

_____

_____

When I was growing up, I loved reading and math in school. I was a shy bespeckled nerd, devouring books and solving number problems. My least favorite subjects were history and social studies. I couldn't see much use in memorizing dates and events. But God had a surprise in store for me. When I went to college, I discovered that history wasn't just about dates and events. It was about people—their interactions with each other and their environments. I began to enjoy stories about people, many who inspired me. I realized that growing up I had relished books about real people, like Annie Sullivan, Helen Keller's teacher, and those books were history. During my second semester of my freshman year, I distinctly heard God calling me to study history. I eventually became a history teacher, sharing my love of history with students and teachers.

David started out as a shepherd but was called to be a king. God's calling in our lives can be to a career choice or service in His church or community that doesn't necessarily start off the way we expect. What is God's calling in your life?

_____

_____

_____

Tanya Murphy from Athens, Tennessee, felt called by God. She had faced difficulties in her life, and God wanted to use her experiences to reach people for Him. His call for her was to load up her car with food and take it to those who were hungry. Her service inspired others, and now the Grace and Mercy Ministries nonprofit includes over fifty churches and crowds of volunteers.[3] Has God used past difficulties in your life to create a passion to serve others in a specific way? If so, how?

_____

_____

_____

God's calling doesn't end after we are established in a career or ministry. God continues to call us throughout our lives. God didn't call me to write Bible studies until I was over 60 years old. Abram answered God's call to go "to the land I will show you" when he was 75 (Genesis 12:1). God called Moses to lead the Israelites out of Egypt when we was 80. Michelangelo painted _The Last Judgment_ on a wall in the Sistine Chapel when he was 89. God has a purpose for you on this earth until the day you leave and enter into His rest. Read and meditate on Isaiah 6:1-8, which is God's calling of the prophet Isaiah. How has God's calling in your life shaped you and impacted others? How do your efforts to make healthy choices in eating and exercise play a part in what God calls you to do?

_____

_____

_____

Thank You, God, for Your calling in my life. I want to be like Isaiah and say, "Here I am; send me" when you call me to missions big and small. Give me Your eyes to see today so I that I am focused on the needs around me and the places You want me to serve in Your Name. Amen.

—— DAY 7: REFLECTION AND APPLICATION

Your love for me is incomprehensible, Lord. You continue to have patience with my stumbling along the way as I take two steps forward and one back in my efforts to put You first and love You with my entire being. Open my heart to hear and prepare me to obey You.

During this first week of studying *Fit for a King*, we have explored God's calling in David's life and our own individual callings from Him, especially in our wellness journeys. He was fit to be king because He was devoted to the one true King. On the seventh day of each week of this study, we will stop and reflect on what God is saying to each of us personally. Your reflections may take one of many forms such as silent prayer, quiet meditation, speaking to God out loud, walking as you communicate with Him, or writing down your thoughts and emotions, just to name a few. You might want to use one of the journaling prompts below to either think or write about these reflections. You do not need to do all of them. Several are listed to give you options from which to choose. There are blank lines at the end of the lesson if you wish to write down anything, or you can use a separate journal.

- **Sketch a large outline of a person's body.** Outside of the body write physical characteristics such as "beautiful hair," "fit figure," and "polished fingernails." On the inside, write the characteristics you have or would like to exemplify that reflect the character of God. You can use scriptures such as Philippians 4:8 and Galatians 5:22-23 for these words. At the bottom of the page, write this week's memory verse, Acts 13:22.
- **Look back at the parts of Psalm 23 from Day 2.** Take each part of the psalm and make it personal. For example, "God, You are my Shepherd, and I have everything I need. You let me rest in green pastures; when I am hungry, You provide me with healthy food that fuels my body to serve you." You can locate or create images that relate to each part of the psalm and include them in your journal.
- **Create a three-column chart.** At the top of each column write one of these phrases from the Day 4 lesson: "Led by God's Spirit," "Ready to Serve," and "Pure in Motive." Under each heading, list examples of each of these parts of God's calling in your life. You can be involved in them now or they may be part of God's work in you for the future.
- **Find a song that encourages you in this reflective process.** You may document the lyrics and record your own reflections on them, or you could illustrate them with sketches or images you locate. Two examples for this week's study are "God Calling" by Jason Reynolds (2020) and "Jesus is Calling" by Vernon Hill (2013).

Your journal holds a very private and personal process; therefore, share it carefully. If social media is a healthy place for you, use these hashtags for posting your words, images, other reflections, or personal stories from this study: #fp4h and #fp4hfitforaking. You can view my journal and others' entries using these hashtags.

As we begin this new study about becoming a person fit for a king, may I pray over us? In the paragraph below, write your name in each blank. Come back to this prayer throughout the study as God calls you to pray for a heart like His that is fit for a king.

Dear Father, _____ is Your child and You have a special calling in _____'s life. You look inside _____ and not at the outside, and You see _____'s unique qualities that You have created in _____. You want to use _____ as a reflection of Your character so that others will see You in _____. This is a high calling, and _____ is ready to follow You and learn more about how _____ can be fit a king. During these next few weeks, help _____ to be focused on You and Your Word, be fervent in prayer, and be faithful to practice the healthy habits You are teaching _____ in First Place for Health. Remove any obstacles that might keep _____ from walking in Your paths of righteousness for Your Name's sake. Protect _____ from the enemy and give _____ the mind of Christ. May everything that _____ does glorify You and draw others closer to You. In Jesus' Name, Amen.

_____

1 Andrew E. Budson, MD, "Why is music good for the brain?" Harvard Health Publishing (2020), https://www. health.harvard.edu/blog/why-is-music-good-for-the-brain-2020100721062.

2 John Schultz, "David, A Man After God's Own Heart," Bible-Commentaries.com (2004), https://www. bible-commentaries.com/source/johnschultz/BC_on-David.pdf.

3 "Three Stories of Service to God," What Does It Mean to Serve God? (2018), https://whatdoesitmeantoserve-god.com/three-stories-of-service-to-god/.

WEEK TWO: DAVID'S FAITH

SCRIPTURE MEMORY VERSE

David said to the Philistine, "You come against me with sword and spear and javelin, but I come against you in the name of the LORD Almighty, the God of the armies of Israel, whom you have defied." 1 Samuel 17:45

David was fit to be Israel's king. He was also called "a man after God's own heart." What does that really mean? One Hebrew scholar describes the phrase this way.

> The phrase *a man after God's own heart* in Hebrew is: *ish kilebabo*. The word *ish* is man, both spiritual and physical. The *ki* is the preposition *like* or *as* and *lebabo* is *his heart*. Tell me, where is the word *after*? You see it? I don't see it. You know why you don't see it, because it is not there. All it says is *a man with a heart like His*. Translators don't like to translate it that way because that is equating us too closely with God, so they paraphrase and say a man *after* God's heart. I used to translate it that way myself until I began my journey to discover the heart of God and when I began to enter God's heart I started to realize that it is possible to have a heart like God's, in fact that is what He is wanting us to have.[1]

Faith is a key ingredient in developing a heart like God's. Do I believe that I can have a heart like God's? And if I do believe, how does God accomplish it in me and what does it look like? If I don't believe, how can God develop my faith so that I fully trust Him? We can learn about living a life of faith by looking at how David believed God throughout many experiences and became a faithful king fit for God's purposes.

Last week in *Fit for a King* we explored David's calling.
- Physical appearances are not God's criteria for His call in people's lives.
- A shepherd's heart protects, provides, and is present for his sheep.
- Music expresses our emotions and can connect all four parts of our being with God's heart.
- A king's heart is led by God's Spirit, ready to serve, and pure in motive.
- We can be confident that God has called us and will walk with us every moment as we seek Him first and learn to love Him with our entire being.

During this week's study we will investigate David's faith, one aspect of his godly heart. Faith is an important part of our wellness journey, too. What we believe about God and ourselves and how we trust Him to make healthy choices contribute to our success in reaching our fitness goals. Like the Hebrew scholar let us commit ourselves to "discover the very heart of God," and as we do, may He continue to make us fit for Him, our mighty King.

—— DAY 1: FAITH TO FACE A GIANT

Today I come to You, my gentle Father, for hope and encouragement. As I encounter the challenges this day brings, may I draw on Your strength and wisdom.

Whenever David's name is mentioned, the first thing that usually comes to mind is his epic battle with Goliath. It was a major step in David's rise to national leadership. At the center is a story of faith in God that inspires us to trust Him when we face our own giants.

To re-familiarize yourself with the story, read 1 Samuel 17. Identify any part of the story that reveals David's faith in God.

_____

_____

_____

After all the time of waiting to see what God would do after He had anointed him, David showed that he was learning how to trust God in the little things. He was ready for this challenge because he had faith in God. What obstacles did he face as he came closer to facing Goliath? First, he had to *overcome enmity*. What did David's brother Eliab say to him in verse 28?

_____

_____

_____

How did David respond (verses 29-30)?

_____

_____

_____

When you are trusting God to bring down the giants in your life, you will often encounter people who will attempt to discourage you. They may be jealous or angry like David's older brother, the one whom Samuel almost anointed before God stopped him (1 Samuel 16:6-7).[2] Even your own family members may be your harshest critics. As you trust God for strength and wisdom in meeting your fitness goals and making healthy choices, you may encounter those who could sabotage your success. As David did, turn away from them and look for encouragement from God and from others who are trusting in Him too.

Next, David had to *overcome expectations*. Read 1 Samuel 17:32-39 and describe King Saul's responses to David's request to fight Goliath (verses 33 and 38).

_____

_____

_____

David knew God had prepared him for this moment. He had proven how he could fight vicious enemies when he saved his sheep from wild animals. He didn't need armor to kill bears and lions with his bare hands. He used a slingshot instead of a sword, which meant he could bring down the giant without hand-to-hand combat, the standard way of fighting. His approach to defeating Goliath went against all expectations for a conquering hero. But David focused on who he was and the unique skills God had developed in him. As you follow Him in your wellness journey, you may find your path looks different from most everyone else. You may lose weight faster or slower than others. You may become stronger in one area before exceling in another. Your faith in God will take you to your goals, and He has promised to complete His good work in you (Philippians 1:6). Trust what He is doing in you and lean into your God-given gifts to conquer your giants.

Finally, David had to *overcome the enemy*. Look at what Goliath said to the Israelites and David in verses 8-10 and 42-44. How would you describe Goliath's words?

_____

_____

_____

This enemy was a real trash talker! Not only did he disparage the Israelites, he even mocked their God. How did the Israelites respond to his ranting (verses 11 and 24)?

_____

_____

_____

Why do you think they responded in this way?

_____

_____

_____

Read David's response to the giant in verses 45-47. Write this week's memory verse here, which is found in this passage.

_____

_____

_____

How is his response different from the other Israelites?

_____

_____

_____

When Goliath defied God and His army, the Israelites saw an insurmountable foe. They shook in their sandals and ran in fear. When David saw Goliath, he saw defiance against his God and boldly stood up for Him. He was confident that God was more powerful than this boastful giant. David spoke boldly to Goliath about the power of his God. We can do the same. No matter what the enemy may throw at us to keep us from following God and making healthy choices we know God is superior. We can speak aloud the Word of God to resist the enemy's attempts to choose less than God's best for us. Our weekly memory verses are weapons we can use in these battles. We face our enemies with God's power, conquering them together with Him. We are fit for a king when we partner with Him to take down giants.

David defeated Goliath because he trusted God. He overcame _enmity, expectations,_ and _enemies._ It is interesting to note that although Goliath was encased in armor from head to toe (verses 5-6), God showed David one weak point: his forehead. That's all it took for his stone to bring down the giant. God gives us ways to overcome what may seem insurmountable odds to reach our fitness goals. We just need to engage with Him in prayer and in His Word. What giants are you facing in your wellness journey right now? Ask God to show you how to overcome the obstacles and put your faith in Him for victory.

_____

_____

_____

Dear Father, You are the giant killer who gives me victory over the enemies that seek to keep me from being fit for a king. I trust You because You love me and You have never failed to keep Your promises. With Your help I am overcoming the obstacles to my fitness goals, and I praise You now for what You are doing in me. Amen.

—— DAY 2: FAITH IN BATTLE
Father, I will face battles in my life today. I do not have the strength to defeat my enemies. But with You I am strong and will conquer every foe. Equip me now for the battles ahead.

Chaplain Carey Cash tells an amazing story about his time serving with the First Battalion, Fifth Marine Regiment during the Iraqi Freedom Mission in 2003. During the forty days before they were to participate in a pivotal battle, Cash led his unit in Bible study. Many churches and families back home were praying for his men and their upcoming conflict. As they marched into Iraq, they saw the hand of God at work, answering their petitions. A line of tanks came out of nowhere but never fired on them. Instead, the unit captured three thousand enemy soldiers who surrendered to them. At the Presidential Palace in Baghdad they encountered an ambush. As one thousand troops fired on them with fifteen hundred rocket-propelled grenades, those in the unit watched in amazement as the grenades sailed around them or fell harmlessly as if "some unseen hand" protected them. One grenade exploded in a Humvee but no soldier died. Chaplain Cash said,

> I remember countless letters I had received from churches saying we are praying specifically when you cross that border that God would restrain and confuse the enemy. The fact that those guns never fired and 3,000 soldiers surrendered en masse tells me God answered the prayer of the people back in the U.S.

Even more incredible are the spiritual victories from this event. Cash's ministry and teaching resulted in sixty Marines accepting Jesus before the battle and a total of 250 people choosing to follow Christ during and after the engagement.[3]

The person fit for a king has faith in God during battles. Some with insurmountable odds. Some with ferocious enemies. Some with long sieges. Some with death and destruction along the way. David faced these circumstances many times in his life. How did faith play a part in his military challenges? Let's start with the time period before David was king. Read 1 Samuel 18:5, 12-16, and 30. Evaluate David's missions and identify how King Saul and the people responded to his leadership.

_____

_____

_____

David's faith in God was evident in his fight with Goliath, but it was not a one-time phenomenon. He trusted God with everything as he faced various enemies on the battlefield. What did that look like practically? We get a glimpse of David's practice in 1 Samuel 23:1-5 and 30:7-8. What do these verses reveal about David's faith, and what was the result of how David responded to threats?

_____

_____

_____

After King Saul was killed in battle, David once again asked God what he should do (2 Samuel 2:1). He asked God for direction, and then he did what God told him to do. This practice sounds so simple, and when David was faithful to follow it, victory was his. How often do I ask and listen to God for direction, whether the situation is seemingly small or large? Do I ask Him daily for His plan for my food and exercise choices? Or do I try my best then later ask Him to bless the good choices and forgive the less healthy ones? As I continue my walk with God, I'm constantly reminded that my continual communication with Him is critical to putting Him first and loving Him with my entire being. I crave the Holy Spirit's leadership and empowerment to walk loyally in His paths for me so I can become fit for Him.

We battle the enemy daily, and he employs spiritual weapons, trying to shoot down our attempts to faithfully follow God. What does 1 Peter 5:8 say about our enemy?

_____

_____

_____

What does verse 9 tell us to do to in order to overcome him?

_____

_____

_____

Whatever battles you face on your wellness journey, you can trust God. He has overcome all the enemies that stand in your way to freedom and fitness through the power of Jesus's death and resurrection. You will see how impotent the enemy becomes in the face of faith in the Father. Write this week's memory verse here and circle the phrase "the Lord Almighty." Faith in Him is your weapon and way to victory.

_____

_____

_____

What battles do you currently face? Tell God about them and thank Him that He is already providing your victory as you learn to trust Him more.

_____

_____

_____

There is nothing I will face today that will surprise You, my Lord. Your power is insurmountable and Your victory is sure. Help me exercise my faith in You, knowing that You can move mountains and calm storms, especially the obstacles that keep me from being free in You. I love You, Father. Amen.

—— DAY 3: FAITH IN TRIALS

The most important part of my day is spending time with You, dear Father. I trust You will open my heart to know You more and build my faith in You, the only wise God and power of the universe.

You might think that after David defeated Goliath, that his life would be great. He would receive praise and accolades, given an exalted spot in the kingdom, and be a trusted confidant of the king. Nothing could be further from the truth. From the time David was victorious over the giant until King Saul's death, he went through severe trials, none of which was his fault. What was the cause of David's suffering? Read 1 Samuel 18:5-9. How did Saul initially treat David after he killed Goliath (verse 5)?

Why did Saul change his attitude toward David (verses 6-9)?

Now read verses 10-11. What did Saul do to David?

Notice the end of verse 11: "But David eluded him twice." Why was there a second attempt? Would you go back after the first one? I don't think I would. David trusted that God would protect him because he was following God's direction. God called him to battle Goliath, and He called him to serve King Saul with his music. But Saul's jealousy caused him to see David as a threat. In fact, Saul tried to kill David many times after these two incidents. But David was faithful to trust God for help. In 1 Samuel 18:12-16, we learn that King Saul sent David away to lead men into battle. What was the result of David's military exploits?

Saul continued to pursue David in order to kill him. Look up 1 Samuel 23:7-14. How did David respond to Saul's attempts to hunt him down?

Putting our faith in God during trials is not easy. When the bills are unpaid, when the illness lingers, when relationships are fractured, we can choose to depend on ourselves to fix the problem. We may isolate and try to find comfort in food. When we do those things, we miss out on the real solution to our trials: resting in God. Proverbs 16:7 says, "When the Lord takes pleasure in anyone's way, he causes their enemies to make peace with them." If we focus on trusting God, He will take care of the rest. It doesn't mean things will be easy, but expending our energy on pursuing God rather than leaning on our own understanding and strength is much easier in the long run.

What trials are you currently facing? How are you trusting God in these trials? Or how did trusting God during a trial in the past turn out for you?

I know I can trust You in the valleys, Lord, for You are ever faithful. As I practice following You with my whole being, strengthen my faith in You. You are greater than whatever trial I face, now and in the future, and I submit to Your gracious wisdom and power. Amen.

—— DAY 4: FAITH IN FRIENDSHIP

Holy Father, still my heart and quiet my mind as I enter into Your awesome presence. May I be open to whatever You have to teach me and let Your Spirit move in me to change me.

Over the decades I have seen many examples of friendship among my fellow First Place for Health members. They pray for each other, contact each other, and minister to each other in practical ways. I remember being in another weight loss program years ago, and although it was a good group, I didn't have the same Christian community I have in First Place for Health. I thrive on the prayers and support I receive from faithful friends who share my desire to follow Christ and my devotion to make healthy choices.

David had a friend who supported him, especially during his most difficult times. That friend was Jonathan, King Saul's son. They first met when David came to the front lines and encountered Goliath. Find 1 Samuel 18:1-4. How does verse 1 describe their relationship?

What actions did Jonathan take in verses 3-4?

_____

_____

_____

Notice verse 2 says that King Saul didn't allow David to return home but that he had to live in the king's courts from that point on. Imagine how David must have felt, forced to leave his home and family, his sheep, and his familiar way of life. He really needed an ally in this foreign setting, especially when King Saul became jealous of him and threw spears at him! Jonathan's friendship must have been a great comfort.

A person fit for kingship knows they cannot be successful alone. They need others to walk alongside them. There are at least three aspects to David and Jonathan's great friendship that connect to our relationships with our First Place for Health members.[4] First, they _sacrificed for each other_. We read that Jonathan gave David his robe, tunic, sword, bow, and belt. These gifts are significant beyond their practical uses. Jonathan was in line to be the next king of Israel after his father died. Somehow Jonathan knew that he would not fill that position but instead David would become king. He graciously stepped aside and supported David's future reign, and he was ready to serve him. He demonstrated humility, both in his friendship with David and his faith in God's plan. As members of a First Place for Health group, we sacrifice our time and attention by engaging with each other: faithfully attending meetings, praying daily for each other, and listening to each other as we make our weekly contacts. Making healthy choices in community is more effective and enjoyable than trying to lose weight by yourself.

Second, David and Jonathan were _loyal to each other and defended each other_. In verse 3 we read that Jonathan made a covenant with David, and they renewed their covenant in 1 Samuel 20:16-17. A covenant was a serious, binding agreement between two or more people that had enormous significance in that culture. It included responsibility for each other's families and financial commitment as if each other's family were their own. Jonathan protected David from his father's murderous anger on more than one occasion. Read 1 Samuel 19:1-7 and describe how Jonathan protected David from his father.

_____

_____

_____

We are loyal to each other in First Place for Health with our positive support in our meetings and our weekly contacts. Our prayers for each other help defend us against the enemy and temptation. We can make healthy choices together at church events by bringing food that fits with our food plan. We can support each other by exercising together. Our loyalty to God and to each other benefits us in all areas of our beings.

Finally, David and Jonathan were *emotionally vulnerable* with each other. They could share their deepest feelings without reserve. We see an example in 1 Samuel 20. King Saul once again planned to kill David but hid his scheme from Jonathan, knowing that he was David's friend. Jonathan discovered his father's intentions and let David know so he could escape. In verses 41 and 42, how do these two friends show their emotional vulnerability to each other as David leaves?

_____

_____

_____

First Place for Health groups provide a safe place for us to express our emotions and be vulnerable. We are all working to eat and exercise in balanced ways through following Jesus. I love to see my group members share their struggles and successes and watch how they support and love on each other. Whether the hugs are physical or virtual, they are life-giving.

David's eulogy after Jonathan died in battle reveals the depth of their friendship. In 2 Samuel 1:26, David says of his dear friend, "I grieve for you, Jonathan my brother; you were very dear to me. Your love for me was wonderful, more wonderful than that of women." How does Proverbs 18:24 describe this kind of friendship?

_____

_____

_____

Faith in a trusted friend is rare, and I thank God for the friends who have supported me throughout my life. Your First Place for Health group is vital to your faith walk and fitness journey. God has provided people to support and love you and for you to love and support in kind. How do your group members faithfully model the aspects of David and Jonathan' friendship?

_____

_____

_____

Thank You for providing the gift of friendship, Lord God. You created humans to be in community with You and with each other, and we need those close relationships to be whole. Bless all our First Place for Health group members as we strive to be faithful friends to each other, seek You first, and love You with all we are. Amen.

—— DAY 5: FAITH IN PROGRESS

Dear Lord, my heart belongs to You. Make me into whatever You have created me to become, and lead me by Your Holy Spirit into the paths You have prepared for me. I want to be fit for a king and serve You well.

We see many examples of David's faith throughout his life's story. In fact he is a member of the Hebrews 11 Hall of Faith, people who demonstrated exemplary trust in God. Look at Hebrews 11:32-34 and notice the list of five other people with whom David is included. Let's take a closer look at two of them and discover why each is listed alongside David as men of great faith.

Gideon (Judges 6:11-8:32)
Background: Gideon was chosen as a judge over Israel. This period of time was between the conquering of the Promised Land and the rule of the kings of Israel, starting with Saul. The Midianites and other foreign armies oppressed the Israelites by invading their land, destroying their crops, and stealing their cattle. As a result, Gideon hid in a wine press threshing his grain, trying to salvage a part of the harvest from the enemies' devastation. This is where we find him in Judges 6:11. An angel appeared to him and gave him a commission in verse 14; what was this commission?

_____

_____

_____

Read Judges 6:36-40. How did Gideon request and get confirmation that God was with him and would bring him victory over the enemy?

_____

_____

_____

A large number of men came out to fight with Gideon, but God reduced the number to only 300 (Judges 7:7). What was the Lord's direction to Gideon to defeat the Midianites (verse 16-18)?

_____

_____

_____

What was the result of Gideon following God's battle plan (verses 21-22)?

_____

_____

_____

Why do you think Gideon is included in the Hebrews 11 Hall of Faith alongside David?

_____

_____

_____

Barak (Judges 4-5)
Background: Barak lived before Gideon during the time of the judges. The Israelites were being oppressed by a Canaanite army led by a cruel general, Sisera. Find Judges 4:4-7. Who was Deborah (verses 4-5)?

_____

_____

_____

What was the commission from God which she gave to Barak (verses 6-7)?

_____

_____

_____

We don't know much about Barak's backstory, but God called him through Deborah to lead the people in battle. What was his response (verse 8)?

_____

_____

_____

What prophesy did Deborah make about Barak (verse 9)?

_____

_____

_____

What was the result of the battle (verse 16)?

_____

_____

_____

Why do you think Barak is included in the Hebrews 11 Hall of Faith alongside David?

_____

_____

_____

One thing that Gideon and Barak shared in common was that they questioned whether or not God was calling them and that He would give them victory. God did not reject them when they doubted or questioned Him but met them where they were. He gave them encouragement through signs and other people so that they grew in their faith and followed Him into battle even when they felt unsure. Gideon went from hiding in a winepress to leading three hundred men against thousands of enemy soldiers, armed only with a jar and a torch. Barak went from seeming obscurity and resistance to leading the Israelites to victory over the Canaanites, helped by two strong women of faith. God uses people from ordinary walks of life whose faith is not yet mature to accomplish amazing things. Wherever you are in your faith development process, God can use you to defeat any enemy. You are ready to conquer your barriers to making consistent healthy choices because you believe in a God Who is the mighty King over all. Even if your faith falters, He will meet you where you are, and He will patiently work in you to accomplish whatever He has planned for you. Your faith makes you fit for a king. Tim Challies writes,

> ...what matters is not the size of a person's faith, but its object. What secures us in our trials is not the magnitude of our faith, but the power of the one in whom we have placed it. The smallest bit of faith in God is worth infinitely more than the greatest bit of faith in ourselves, or the strongest measure of faith in faith itself. Faith counts for nothing unless its object is Jesus Christ.[5]

I trust You, Father, for every breath I take and every step I make. I am nothing without You. As I learn to trust You more, show me Your power and might while I seek You first and love You with all my being. Amen.

—— DAY 6: REFLECTION AND APPLICATION

I stand in awe of Your amazing love and grace, dear Lord. Every day You are with me, never leaving me alone and constantly calling me into a deeper walk with You. I'm ready to listen to You now.

Practice this week's memory verse.

_____

_____

_____

Physical and mental illnesses are formidable giants. When a loved one has cancer, when a child has an emotional disorder, when a friend is dying, we may feel helpless. We fall to our knees and plead with God for healing and strength. Paul encourages us to "pray without ceasing" (1 Thessalonians 5:17 NASB), and James 5:15 tells us that the prayer offered in faith can heal. Jesus encountered a father who wanted Him to heal his son. His condition caused him to be mute, throw himself to the ground, foam at the mouth, and become rigid. Read Mark 9:21-24. What did the father say to Jesus in verse 22?

_____

_____

_____

What was Jesus' response in verse 23?

_____

_____

_____

What did the father request in verse 24?

_____

_____

_____

Jesus healed the boy. I would imagine the father's faith was strengthened after that miraculous experience! It's a bit of a paradox: we learn to trust God more by trusting Him and experiencing His answers to our prayers. God helps us with our unbelief by asking us to believe He can do impossible things then showing us He can. It's like a muscle; the more we exercise it, the stronger it gets. Read Luke 18:27 and write it here.

_____

_____

_____

Chuck Swindoll says that we are constantly faced with "great opportunities brilliantly disguised as impossible situations."[6] What impossible thing are you trusting God to do? Or is there an impossible situation that you need to trust God to do?

_____

_____

_____

How can this be an opportunity for your faith to grow?

_____

_____

_____

Let's end our reflection today with some of David's words of faith from the Psalms.

> When I am afraid, I put my trust in you. In God, whose word I praise—in God I trust and am not afraid. What can mere mortals do to me? In God, whose word I praise, in the Lord, whose word I praise—in God I trust and am not afraid. What can can do to me? (Psalm 56:3-4, 10-11)

Stepping out in faith can be scary, Lord, but I know You never disappoint those who trust in You and obey Your direction. Help my unbelief and show me where I need to fully trust You. You are mighty to save and full of grace and mercy; what can I fear when I am in Your care? Amen.

—— DAY 7: REFLECTION AND APPLICATION

My hope is built on You alone, my dear Father God. I can trust nothing else on this earth with all of myself. Your promises are powerful and Your presence is peaceful.

David's biblical saga has much to teach us about faith in God and how it made him fit to be Israel's king. No matter what event or enemy we face, God is able to conquer it. When we are on His side, the battle is already won. As you reflect on God's Word today, ask Him to show you His power and might in challenges that require faith in Him. Below are some possible prompts for meditation and journaling. Remember, you don't need to do them all. These are just suggestions to spark your thoughts and connect you more deeply to God.

- **In the middle of a journal page, write "My Battles" and circle it.** Draw lines from the circle out to the edges of the page. On each line write a scripture reference that encourages you in fighting your battles with God's help. Some examples include 1 Peter 5:8-9 and Romans 8:37.
- **Contact a friend who encourages you**, either in your First Place for Health group or someone else. You can text, call, or write to your friend. Tell them how their friendship impacts your life and how much you appreciate their faithfulness. Share what God is doing in your life presently and ask how you can pray for them. Record your thoughts about this conversation in your journal.
- **Make a two-column chart.** Title the first column "Fear" and the second column "Faith." Make a list of things that cause you to be afraid in the first column. In the second column, list ways that God has shown you that you have nothing to fear when He is with you. You can include scripture verses such as Psalm 56:3-4 and 10-11.
- **Find a song that encourages you** in this reflective process. You may document the lyrics and record your own reflections on them, or you could illustrate them with sketches or images you locate. Two examples for this week's study are "Confidence" by Sanctus Real (2018) and "Stand in Faith" by Danny Gokey (2021).

Your journal holds a very private and personal process; therefore, share it carefully. If social media is a healthy place for you, use these hashtags for posting your words, images, other reflections, or personal stories from this study: #fp4h and #fp4hfitforaking. You can view my journal and others' entries using these hashtags.

I believe You are the God of David, the one and only God of the universe, creator, sustainer, savior, and king. Help me to trust You in all things, knowing that You always have my best at the heart of all You do. Thank You for saving me and making me Your cherished child. I love You. Amen.

_____

1 Chaim Bentorah, "Word Study–A Heart Like God's" Chaim Bentorah's Daily Word Study (2015), https://www.chaimbentorah.com/2015/08/word-study-a-heart-like-gods-%D7%99%D7%94%D7%95%D7%94-%D7%9B%D7%9C%D7%91%D7%91%D7%95/.

2 Beth Moore, David: 90 Days with a Heart Like His (Nashville: BH Publishing Group, 2006), 77.

3 John Livingston Clark, "War Stories of Divine Intervention," The Bottom Line (2014), https://www.tblfaithnews.com/featured/war-stories-of-divine-intervention.

4 "What Was the Relationship between David and Jonathan?" Got Questions, https://www.gotquestions.org/David-and-Jonathan.html.

5 Tim Challies, "What Matters is Not the Size of Your Faith," Challies (2021), https://www.challies.com/articles/what-matters-is-not-the-size-of-your-faith/.

6 Charles Swindoll, "The Astonishing Power of Jesus," Insight for Living (2024), https://insight.org/broadcasts/player/?bid=4634.

WEEK THREE: DAVID'S WORSHIP

SCRIPTURE MEMORY VERSE
Come, let us sing to the Lord! Let us shout joyfully to the Rock of our salvation. Let us come to him with thanksgiving. Let us sing psalms of praise to him.
Psalm 95:1-2 (NLT)

What do you think of when you hear the word *worship*? You may picture going to church on Sunday morning, participating in a gathering where music and preaching are present. Although attending corporate worship services is an essential part of a Christian's practice, it is not the essence of the meaning of worship. Music is an integral part of many worship services, but it is an expression of worship, not worship itself. Emotion can follow acts of worship, but it also is not what worship means. In the Hebrew Bible the main word used for worship is *shachah*, and it means "depress," "bow down," or "prostrate." This word creates an image of falling down before God in awe and respect. "The Old Testament idea is therefore the reverential attitude of mind or body or both, combined with the more generic notions [about] adoration, obedience, [and] service."[1] The Greek word used most often in the New Testament is *proskuneō* and has a similar meaning. When we encounter God and we recognize His supremacy and sovereignty and respond with humility and affection, we participate in worship.

David is often depicted in a worshiping posture . Sometimes he physically prostrated himself before God, displaying either great love or crushing remorse. One of the reasons he is described as "a man after God's own heart" and was fit for a king is that his heart was full of worship for the Lord. He gave credit to God for all of his accomplishments and was grateful for all God's blessings, often saying that he and his family were unworthy of what God had done for them. His life is an example of how to worship God consistently and reverently.

Last chapter in *Fit for a King* we explored David's faith.
- In order to conquer our giants, we may need to overcome enmity, expectations, and the enemy as we trust in God.
- Faith in God can help us overcome insurmountable odds as God defeats our enemies through His power and might.

- We can trust God even during trials and find rest in Him.
- Faithful friends like David and Jonathan sacrifice for each other, are loyal and defend each other, and are emotionally vulnerable with each other.
- God will meet us where we are in our faith journey; a small amount of faith in the mighty God can accomplish great things.

This week we will look at David's heart and practice of worship. We can learn how to worship God daily in our fitness journey, constantly involving Him in our decisions to make healthy choices and giving Him His proper place as King on the throne of our hearts.

—— DAY 1: WORSHIP WITH ABANDON

I worship You, Lord, with my whole heart, opening myself to Your marvelous presence. I bow down to You, my Maker and Savior, for You the King are worthy of all praise and worship.

Write this week's memory verse here.

_____

_____

_____

What is your worship style? You may sit or stand in silence with your head bowed. You may raise your hands. You may move your body. You may do different things at different times. These are all reactions to the act of worshipping our great God. But what does it mean to authentically worship God? David shows us an example in a story from 1 Chronicles. Read chapter 15, verses 1 and 3 to get some background.

The ark of the covenant had been away from the tabernacle for many years after being captured by the Philistines in a battle. It was an essential part of Israel's worship of God, representing the holiest spot where He met with His people. David wanted to bring it back to its proper place and now was the time. He had become ruler of all of Israel, and it was one of the first things he did as king. Verses 4-15 tell about David's preparations for bringing the ark into Jerusalem. What plan did he make in verse 16?

_____

_____

_____

Other people who were involved in the proceedings are listed in verses 17-24. In verse 25 the festivities began. Fill in the details below.

Verse 25: "...bring up the ark of the covenant . . . with _____."

Verse 26: "Because God had helped the Levites who were carrying the ark of the covenant of the Lord _____ _____ and _____ _____ were _____."

Verse 27: "David was clothed in a robe of _____ _____."

Verse 28: "So all Israel brought up the ark of the covenant of the Lord with _____, with the sounding of rams' _____ and _____, and of _____, and the playing of _____ and _____."

Verse 29 tells us that David was dancing and celebrating before the Lord as well.

This worship event included joyful attitudes, animal sacrifices, priestly garments, music, shouting, dancing, and celebrating. The Israelites worshipped with abandon! David and his people could barely contain themselves because they were very excited about bringing the ark of the covenant back to its rightful place in the tabernacle. It represented the presence of God and all He had done to make Israel His people, despite their unfaithfulness over the years. David and the people held nothing back as they expressed their reverence to God, their gratitude for His care for them, and their joy at the return of the ark. Their desire to show and tell God that they respected Him and wanted to serve Him is at the heart of real worship. They expressed that desire in many ways. But if their hearts were not authentically bowed before God in reverence, the ceremony would have been empty ritual. "True worship is the result of conviction, affection, and truth."[2] Emotion and physical responses may result from worship because our entire beings are focused on God and loving Him.

Let's look at three stories from the New Testament that exemplify worshipping God with abandon. How did each of these people express authentic worship?

The widow in Mark 12:41-44

_____

_____

_____

The woman with Jesus in Luke 7:36-50

_____

_____

_____

Paul and Silas in Acts 16:23-25

_____

_____

_____

Like these people, we can choose to let go of our struggles and worship with abandon. We can choose to put aside our desire to make independent decisions in our eating and exercise routines and instead focus all our attention on Him. When Jesus triumphantly entered Jerusalem on a donkey on what we call Palm Sunday, He said "if [the people] keep quiet, the stones will cry out" (Luke 19:40). The people laid their robes and palm branches down for Him to welcome Him into the city as their king. They didn't hold anything back as they shouted, "Hosanna!" "Blessed is he who comes in the name of the Lord!" (John 12:13). When we are authentically engaged in worship with our Lord, we cannot contain ourselves. It may look like energetic singing or quiet surrender, but the common denominator is complete surrender to God. What is one thing you will do today to worship Him with abandon?

_____

_____

_____

How I love You, Lord! I want to release my desires for unhealthy and selfish choices and replace them with a heart that yearns to worship You. Help me walk in worship all day as I praise and honor You with everything I do. Amen.

—— DAY 2: WORSHIP IN HIS PRESENCE

Oh Father, my life is full of challenges and commitments. I put them all aside right now to spend time with You, my loving Lord. Speak Your truth to me now.

There are many interesting sites to see in the big state of Texas. A popular tour-ist attraction in the area around Schulenberg is the Painted Churches Tour. More than 20 churches were built in the late 1800s and early 1900s by Czech and Ger-man immigrants who wanted to incorporate some of their native culture in their new communities in Texas. The churches contain awe-inspiring art and architec-ture, pointing us to God and inviting us to come into His presence to worship Him.

David desperately wanted to build a house for God. In 2 Samuel 7 he told the proph-et Nathan about his plans, but God replied through Nathan that David would not be the one to build the temple. Read 1 Chronicles 28:2-3; what did David say about his desire to construct a house for God?

_____

_____

_____

The tabernacle in Jerusalem, which was replaced by the temple, was a sacred place where God's presence came to meet with His people. It had been the place for the Israelites to worship God since He gave them the plans at Mount Sinai (Exodus 26). Although David didn't get to build the temple, he did everything he could to prepare for its construction by his son Solomon, the heir to his throne, who took his father's plans and created a spectacular structure for the worship of God (1 Kings 5-8).

Why was David consumed by a desire to build a house for God, a place to encounter His presence and worship Him? Let's look at one of his prayers recorded in Psalms to get some insight. Read Psalm 42:1-3. How does David express his need for God?

_____

_____

_____

Now read verse 4. What is David remembering and how does he feel?

_____

_____

_____

What memory or memories do you have of spending time in church that are most meaningful to you?

_____

_____

_____

David wrote this psalm when he was forced to flee into the wilderness away from Jerusalem. Imagine David's passionate longing to be in God's presence and worship Him in the tabernacle, seen in this psalm and many other times in the Bible. His worship of God seemed to be more important to him than any other desire, including physical sustenance. Although he could and did worship God in His presence in other locations, that sacred tabernacle connected him with God in a way no other place could.

I am challenged by David's yearning to be in God's presence. Do I desire God more than I desire anything, including food? What if I sacrificed my desires for food, laid them all on the altar, and allowed God to make all decisions about food for me? What if I looked at eating as a way to worship God my King, to be fully surrendered to His sovereignty? Planning meals and making healthy choices can be expressions of worship to the God I revere and adore by submitting to His authority and obeying His Word. We don't have to go to a temple to enter into God's presence any more. My body is the temple of the Holy Spirit, the place where God has chosen to put His presence on earth. I am His sacred place, and I want to hunger for Him more than anything else. It is easy to worship God with praise music on Sunday, but it is harder to worship Him Monday through Saturday by following His Spirit's direction and putting healthy habits into practice. What do your food and exercise choices reveal about your desire for God?

_____

_____

_____

Entering into God's presence to worship and praise Him is experiencing some of heaven, where we will live in God's presence forever. It allows God to transform us from the inside out and gives us the opportunity to express our love and gratitude to Him. Let's end our quiet time with Him today by meditating on part of David's prayer as the plans for the temple were finalized and he handed the project over to Solomon. Read 1 Chronicles 29:10-13 and make it your own prayer as you worship God in His presence.

Praise be to you, LORD, the God of our father Israel, from everlasting to everlasting. Yours, LORD, is the greatness and the power and the glory and the majesty and the splendor, for everything in heaven and earth is yours. Yours, LORD, is the kingdom; you are exalted as head over all. Wealth and honor come from you; you are the ruler of all things. In your hands are strength and power to exalt and give strength to all. Now, our God, we give you thanks, and praise your glorious name.

Holy Father, I long to abide in Your presence all week and all day long. In Your presence I find peace, hope, and strength that I don't have on my own. May my thoughts and actions today reflect my adoration of You and my deep desire to worship and honor You. Amen.

—— DAY 3: WORSHIP AS CONVERSATION

I worship You, O Lord, for You are worthy of all praise and honor. You are above all powers and all things, majestic and holy, Creator of all I see. I bow before You now as I seek Your face.

Yesterday we used a prayer of David's to end our study time. According to the Bible his life was filled with prayer. He spoke to God when he was happy, sad, and angry and when he needed help or forgiveness. Prayer was an integral part of His worship and adoration of God. At its heart prayer is conversation with God. It is listening to Him as well as talking with Him. As we come into His presence, bowing in awe and respect, we hear His Word and respond with our thoughts and feelings. It reflects our personal connection with Him as we commune with the One Who created us for relationship.

Read Psalm 55:17. What does this verse indicate about the frequency of David's prayers?

_____

_____

_____

We can imagine David in perpetual prayer mode, listening and speaking to God non-stop. And regardless of the circumstance, he was transparent before God. Look up each of the following verses and identify what David said that reveals his openness before Him.

Scripture	How David Was Open with God
Psalm 55:4-5	
Psalm 51:4	
Psalm 139:19-22	

Psalm 13 is another example of David conversing authentically with God. What do verses 1-2 tell us about David's state of mind?

_____

_____

_____

What does he ask God to do in verses 3-4?

_____

_____

_____

How does he end his conversation with God in verses 5-6?

_____

_____

_____

What can we learn about prayer from David, the man after God's heart who was fit to be Israel's king? People who follow David's example talk to God twenty-four/seven, not just at church, before meals, during their quiet time, or when they need help. Their prayers are not just lists of petitions but true conversation with God, a two-way street. They lay everything on the table, holding nothing back. They crave talking with God just as someone with a new love interest can't wait to talk with them about their day and how they feel about them.

Prayer is an imperative practice in First Place for Health. We talk with God about our emotional, spiritual, mental, and physical status and ask Him for direction in making healthy choices. Being engaged with Him gives us power to overcome temptation and receive the victories He has prepared for us. We gain wisdom and perspective. How does your prayer life represent this kind of conversation with God?

_____

_____

_____

Take a moment to write a prayer to God modeled on Psalm 8. First, tell God about your current state of mind.

_____

_____

_____

Then ask Him for help where needed.

_____

_____

_____

Finally, express praise and adoration for the God Who hears your prayers and loves you beyond understanding.

_____

_____

_____

Now take time for an important part of prayer: stop and *listen* to God. We are often quick to talk to God and then go on our way without waiting to hear His voice. You may or may not sense a reply at this moment, but continue to listen to Him concerning the prayer you wrote. When you do hear from Him, how did He respond?

_____

_____

_____

Worshipping God like David involves intimate, authentic prayer, conversing with God consistently throughout each day. Meditate on these ideas about prayer and explore how God wants to commune with you more deeply.

Precious Lord, I have so much to say to You, to tell You my heart's deepest desires and concerns. Thank You that You always listen to me and answer my prayers. Help me to listen to You more closely and walk in prayer with You throughout this day. I love You. Amen.

—— DAY 4: WORSHIP IN REVERENCE

O Lord, our Lord, how majestic is Your Name in all the earth! You are the only wise God, and I bow before You now in worship, recognizing Your holiness and supremacy.

Author Philip Yancey shared an experience he had while traveling in Alaska.

> Against the slate-gray sky, the water of an ocean inlet had a slight greenish cast, interrupted by small whitecaps. Soon I saw these were not whitecaps at all, but whales—silvery white beluga whales in a pod feeding no more than fifty feet offshore. I stood with the other onlookers for forty minutes, listening to the rhythmic motion of the sea, following the graceful, ghostly crescents of surfacing whales. The crowd was hushed, even reverent. For just that moment, nothing else—dinner reservations, the trip schedule, life back home—mattered. We were confronted with a scene of quiet beauty and a majesty of scale. We felt small. We strangers stood together in silence until the whales moved farther out. Then we climbed the bank together and got in our cars to resume our busy, ordered lives that suddenly seemed less urgent.[3]

Yancey's story expresses an experience of awe and reverence. Can you remember a time when you felt this way? What were the circumstances and the impact on you?

_____

_____

_____

It is possible that the onslaught of media we experience every day has dulled our sense of reverence and awe. That is unfortunate, because feeling awe is actually good for us. According to a 2018 study, "Awe [makes] us see ourselves as a small piece of something larger." You may have more positive thoughts than negative ones and have a greater sense of well-being.[4] David recorded many expressions of awe that were inspired by God and His creation. Let's look at Psalm 8, verses 1 and 9. How did David start and end this psalm?

_____

_____

_____

Verses 1 and 2 provide a contrast between two ways God's majesty is described: His glory in the heavens, which is great, and the speech of babies, which is small. In verses 3-4, what did David observe that caused him to revere God?

_____

_____

_____

How did he describe human beings in verses 5-8?

_____

_____

_____

David had the proper perspective of humans in relationship to God in this psalm. God our King is great beyond our comprehension. The world would have us believe that we are the center of the universe, that we are all powerful and deserve the best of everything. But if we withdraw from life's hustle and consider the majesty and glory of God, evident all around us, we know that viewpoint is false. And when we seek to worship God, we must view Him as the One above all.

Many times we read "the fear of God" in the Bible, as in Deuteronomy 10:12. It is important to know that "fear" in this context is not fear of something bad happening but deep submission and reverence, understanding He is supreme, mighty, and inscrutable. If you entered into the presence of a world leader, you would feel a sense of awe and respect, just because of who they are and their high-ranking office. Being in God's presence evokes an even greater sense of awe. What does the first part of Proverbs 1:7 tell us about the "fear of the Lord"?

_____

_____

_____

Reverencing God leads us to understand who He is and who we are in relationship to Him. Read Hebrews 12:28; how are we instructed to worship God?

_____

_____

_____

The difference between being afraid of God and being in awe of God depends on your status before God. God's holy presence is frightening to someone who doesn't know and have a relationship with Him through Jesus His Son. God's holy presence is dangerous to those who have not received His righteousness through Jesus's spilt blood on the cross. If we have been "born again" (John 3) and choose to follow Jesus, we are not in danger when we come into His holy presence. What does Hebrews 4:16 say?

_____

_____

_____

If you haven't yet accepted God's gracious gift of salvation through Jesus, you may feel more fear than awe. Ask God to forgive your sin and receive life through Him. Talk to your First Place for Health leader about the opportunity to know God through Jesus's sacrifice for you. You will know the One Who created everything including you, and as His child, you will experience awe and wonder in worshipping Him.

Lord, our Lord, how majestic is Your name in all the earth! I am awestruck when I think about the complexity of the universe and the way You work in my life every day. You are King of all things, and I'm so grateful You are Lord of my life. Amen.

—— DAY 5: WORSHIP TO KNOW GOD

I come to You, Lord, hungry for Your presence. I desire to know You more than anything, and I want to hear You speak to me in new and fresh ways as I worship You now.

David, the man after God's heart, craved God deeply. Many times in his prayers recorded in the Psalms, he cries out to Him with an overwhelming desire to know his King more intimately. Read Psalm 63:1-2. How did David describe his yearning for God?

_____

_____

_____

Fill in the blanks below with David's expressions of worship found in verses 2-4.

I have seen you in the _____ and beheld your _____ and your

_____.

Because your _____ is better than _____, my _____

will _____ you.

I will _____ you as long as I _____ , and in your _____
I will _____ _____ my _____ .

In verse 5 David compares being satisfied with God to another type of satisfaction; what is it?

_____
_____
_____

Worshipping God can fill me up in ways that food never can. Each of us has an empty spot inside of us that only God can fill. If you struggle with binge eating, emotional eating, or mindless eating, it might be a sign that you are hungry for something other than physical food. Look up Romans 14:17 and fill in the blanks below.

The kingdom of God is not _____ .

The kingdom of God is _____ .

Read Isaiah 55:1-2. What does God call us to do?

_____
_____
_____

What does He encourage us to do in verse 6?

_____
_____
_____

Spending time in God's presence, worshipping and experiencing Him, is immensely satisfying. Perhaps I need to turn my attention to worshipping God when I am tempted to gratify a craving with an unhealthy choice. It is hard to put food in my mouth and sing praises to God at the same time! Find Psalm 19:9-10. What is pure and endures forever?

_____
_____
_____

What qualities of God's decrees are listed in these verses? There are at least four.

_____

_____

_____

Maybe the cure for my sweet tooth is to find sweetness in God, His presence, and His Word. I want to know Him more, and in Him I will find the answer to my hungers. How much do you want to know God and how does that desire influence your worship of Him?

_____

_____

_____

Turn to God in worship this week when you are tempted to make a less than healthy choice. He is truly all we need.

I find satisfaction in You alone, Lord, my maker and my God. Fill me with You so that I crave nothing else. Turn me away from things that keep me from growing in my knowledge of You, and help me to walk in Your life-giving presence every step of my daily walk. Amen.

—— DAY 6: REFLECTION AND APPLICATION

I bring my heart to You, my Father, and ask You to take it for Your own. I give up my selfish agenda and distracted mind so I can know You in this quiet time of worship and reflection.

Practice reciting this week's memory verses here.

_____

_____

_____

These verses were written by David and indicate that he was one of God's biggest fans! At the beginning of this week, we looked at his desire to build the temple and God's plan for his son Solomon to build it instead. David worshipped and praised God after learning this news. Read 2 Samuel 7:22-24. How did David praise God?

_____

_____

_____

David sacrificed his own desire to construct God's temple and praised Him for His promises for His people past, present, and future. He brought a sacrifice of praise, honoring God and His plans rather than himself and his own plans. When the Israelites participated in worship, they always brought a sacrifice.

> They never came empty-handed, believing that by giving something to the divine, they could invite blessings and favor in return. These prayers and offerings were often made before important events such as harvests, births, or weddings as a way to seek divine protection and blessings. The underlying principle was that if you wanted to ask something of your gods, you needed to give something in return. The God of Israel was no different in this respect. Do you wish to meet and ask of Him something? Great! But lunch is on you, so don't forget to prepare and bring a nice "meal" with you when you come to the altar.[5]

Fortunately, as believers in Christ, we do not have to adhere to the sacrificial rituals of the Mosaic covenant. Jesus became our sacrifice through His death on the cross and no further blood sacrifice is needed (Hebrews 7:27). But we want to worship God our King reverently and authentically. When we worship God, what do we bring to Him? What do we sacrifice so that we can honor Him and know Him more? Some Christians put this idea into practice every year at Lent, the forty days prior to Easter. It connects them to the forty days that Jesus fasted in the wilderness after his baptism and before He began His public ministry (Matthew 4). During Lent you give up something important to you, such as food or an activity, or you devote a specific time to God each day.

What does Hebrews 13:15-16 tell us about sacrifice?

_____

_____

_____

> "The command in Hebrews 13:15 says that this sacrifice is to be offered 'continually.' Our praise of God is not to be based on our opinion of His job performance. Praise cannot be treated as a 'reward' we give God for His obvious blessings."[6]

We praise God for Who He is: compassionate and gracious, slow to anger, abounding in loyal love and faithfulness (Exodus 34:6). Consider your experience of worship, both corporately and individually. How do you praise God during these times?

_____

_____

_____

How does your praise represent personal sacrifice?

_____

_____

_____

Psalm 25 starts out with a great song of praise to God. But when you look at the context of the psalm, you find that David was going through a rough patch. Sometimes our sacrifice of praise means praising God during difficult times. We sacrifice our need to focus on ourselves and what we don't have and instead choose to focus on God and Who He is. We lay all our hurts and pains at His feet and worship Him with grateful hearts, trusting that He will be all we need. Have you ever praised God in the midst of trials? If so, what did you do? If not, what could you do?

_____

_____

_____

In John 4:24, Jesus told the Samaritan woman at the well that "God is spirit, and his worshipers must worship in the Spirit and in truth." His Spirit lives within us, and His Word is truth. We praise Him for these gifts. And it is only through His Spirit and His Word that we are transformed from the inside out to live a life of healthy choices. How can you worship God in spirit and in truth through your fitness journey?

_____

_____

_____

Praise God from Whom all blessings flow. Praise Him, all creatures here below. Praise Him above, ye heavenly host. Praise Father, Son, and Holy Ghost. Praise God, Who is worthy of all praise, honor, and glory. Amen.

—— DAY 7: REFLECTION AND APPLICATION

As I step away from the world and into Your presence, Lord, I need to hear Your voice and know Your mind. See my desire to find all I need in You and fill my longings.

This week we have explored David's life of worship and considered our own worship practices. As you spend time today reflecting on what God is saying to you, include time to worship Him in ways that reveal your heart for Him. Here are some ideas you may choose to use in that process.

- **Record words and/or images that express worshipping God** with abandon. One example would be an image of someone raising their hands in a worship service. Another example would be writing verses from the Bible that express joyful worship such as additional verses from Psalm 25.
- **Take a worship walk.** If you are outdoors you can identify things in nature that glorify God's creativity and power. If you are indoors you can use scripture, praise music, images of nature, or your own words to tell God how much He means to you.
- **In the middle of a journal page sketch a table or altar.** Above the altar list things that you want to sacrifice to God, including food that is not healthy for you or a habit that keeps you from fully engaging with Him. Below the altar write a prayer of commitment to Him that indicates you will choose worshipping Him over the things you have written on the altar.
- **Find a song that encourages you in this reflective process.** You may document the lyrics and record your own reflections on them, or you could illustrate them with sketches or images you locate. Two examples for this week's study are "Completely Abandoned" by Gateway Worship (2023) and "Sing for Joy" by Don Moen (2000).

Your journal holds a very private and personal process; therefore, share it carefully. If social media is a healthy place for you, use these hashtags for posting your words, images, other reflections, or personal stories from this study: #fp4h and #fp4hfitforaking. You can view my journal and others' entries using these hashtags.

I want to worship You, Lord, because of Who You are and how much You mean to me. May my life reflect a heart like Yours as I walk in worship and praise of my mighty King and loving Lord. I love You. Amen.

1 "Worship," Bible Hub, https://biblehub.com/topical/w/worship.htm.

2 "What is true worship?" Got Questions, https://www.gotquestions.org/true-worship.html.

3 "A Moment of Wonder in Alaska's Wilderness," Christianity Today/Preaching Today, https://www.preachingtoday.com/illustrations/2016/march/7032116.html.

4 Sarah DiGiulio, "Why Scientists Say Experiencing Awe Can Help You Live Your Best Life," Better by Today (2019), https://www.nbcnews.com/better/lifestyle/why-scientists-say-experiencing-awe-can-help-you-live-your-ncna961826.

5 Eitan Bar, "Hebrew Word Study – Shachah," Eitan Bar, https://eitan.bar/articles/hebrew-word-study-worship-shachah/.

6 "What Does It Mean to Give a Sacrifice of Praise? (Hebrews 13:15)" Got Questions, https://www.gotquestions.org/sacrifice-of-praise.html.

WEEK FOUR: DAVID'S SONGS

SCRIPTURE MEMORY VERSE
Sing to the Lord a new song; sing to the Lord, all the earth. Sing to the Lord, praise his name; proclaim his salvation day after day. Declare his glory among the nations, his marvelous deeds among all peoples. Psalm 96:1-3

Music fills my days. When I get into my car, I immediately turn on some music. When I'm feeling blue, I play music that lifts my mood. When I spend time alone with God, I enjoy singing and listening to my favorite hymns and praise music. I sing in my church choir. My grandson and I love to listen to Disney tunes in the car. I love all kinds of music: Christian, show tunes, rock and roll, classical, and jazz, just to name a few. And through various apps, I can access any kind of music I desire anytime and anywhere.

David was a musician, and his music fills the pages of the Bible. Most of his songs are recorded in the book of Psalms. Almost half of the chapters are attributed to him: 73 out of 150. "The Hebrew word for psalm, *mizmôr*, means 'melody.' You won't find this word anywhere else in the Bible—only in the titles of the Psalms."[1] Although he was a rugged warrior and powerful ruler, the heart of this king was full of songs for his God. "David was always translating his daily experience into songs and prayers of faith."[2]

For last week's *Fit for a King* we studied David's worship.
- Worshipping with abandon involves letting go of my struggles and focusing completely on God.
- Yearning to be in God's presence calls me to worship Him and desire Him above everything else.
- Praying is part of worship and involves conversation with God, including listening to Him.
- Respecting God leads us to understand who He is and who we are in relationship to Him.
- Worshipping God fills my desire to know Him, an innate longing that only He can satisfy.

This week we will enjoy meditating on some of the psalms of David. The man fit to be Israel's king wrote songs that call us to God and speak of His love for us. Music plays a powerful role in our relationship to God. We connect with Him through melody and lyrics, expressing our emotions and devotion, impacting each of the four parts of our beings as we focus our lives on Him.

—— DAY 1: PRAISE

Bless the Lord, oh my soul! My entire being praises You, mighty God, my Father and Lord. Fill my heart with a new song as I enter into Your presence with praise.

Write this week's memory verses here.

_____

_____

_____

There is not a specific section in the Psalms that contains all the praise songs and prayers. "The entire book of Psalms is called 'psalm of praise' in the Hebrew Bible."[3] Words that celebrate the majesty and glory of God run throughout the entire book. David habitually praised God, and one of his greatest praise songs is Psalm 103. Let's dive into this psalm by reading verses 1-2. What did David want to remember about God?

_____

_____

_____

Why do you suppose David repeated the phrase "praise (bless) the Lord, oh my soul" in these two verses?

_____

_____

_____

What are the benefits of God that he recalled in verses 3-5?

Who _____ all your _____

And _____ all your _____

Who _____ your _____ from the _____

And _____ you with _____ and _____

Who _____ your _____ with _____ _____

So that your _____ is _____ like the _____

Why do you think we should we remember these benefits of God?

For what does David praise God in verse 6?

Read verses 8-12. What characteristics of God does David list in verses 8-9?

How does God handle our sin in verses 10-12?

Verses 13 and 17-18 are bookends for the next section of this psalm. What does David say about God in these verses?

In verses 14-16 David describes our nature. What does he say about human beings?

How do verses 13 and 17-18 relate to verses 14-16?

In verse 19, David reminds us of the grandeur of God: "The Lord has established his throne in heaven, and his kingdom rules over all." Then he ends the psalm by calling others to join in his praise for God. Who are they?

Verse 20 _____

Verse 21 _____

Verse 22 _____

Then he ends the psalm with one last enthusiastic call to "Praise the Lord, my soul." What are your thoughts and feelings after reading through this psalm of praise?

_____

_____

_____

Praising God is applauding Him for all He is and does. I praise Him because He is loving, merciful, and gracious. I praise Him for never leaving me alone. I praise Him because He has brought me through enormous difficulties. I praise Him for healing my brokenness. He deserves all my praise, and when I stand and lift my hands to Him, I'm giving Him a standing ovation. How can you applaud God today?

_____

_____

_____

How does praising God impact your faith walk and wellness journey?

_____

_____

_____

Praise You, loving Lord and Creator of all the universe. Praise You for Your amazing power, the sacrifice of Jesus, and the indwelling of Your Holy Spirit. Praise the Lord, my soul! Amen.

—— DAY 2: SONG

Be exalted, O God, above the heavens and let Your glory be over all the earth! Fill my heart with songs of praise to You, and encourage me with Your Word.

When I was growing up, my two sisters and I took turns doing the dinner dishes in pairs. While two of us washed, rinsed, dried, and put away the dishes, we would often sing. Show tunes were a staple of our repertoire, especially "Oklahoma!" and "The Sound of Music," two of my mom's favorites. It made a daily chore much more enjoyable. Music provides many benefits, psychologically and physiologically. It can decrease pain and anxiety. It can help memory retention and alleviate stress. It is even used in treating brain injuries and seizures.[4] Although David was unaware of the science behind music's advantages, he knew what it did for him and his relationship with God. Look up Psalm 108. What does David say in verse 1?

_____

_____

_____

When and where is David singing in verses 2-3?

_____

_____

Why is David singing to God (verse 4)?

_____

_____

What does David sing to God in verse 5?

_____

_____

_____

Many of our contemporary praise and worship songs come directly from David's psalms.[5] Let's look at some examples. Read Psalm 27:1-3, an inspiration for Chris Tomlin's "Whom Shall I Fear (God of Angel Armies)." How does David describe God in verse 1?

_____

_____

_____

What does God do for David in verses 2-3?

_____

_____

_____

Another example of David's psalms inspiring contemporary Christian music is "My Soul Will Wait (Psalm 62)" by Sovereign Grace. Find Psalm 62:5-8. What does David find in God in verse 5?

_____

_____

_____

What metaphors does David use to describe God in verses 6-7?

_____

_____

_____

What does David encourage us to do in verse 8?

_____

_____

_____

Finally, let's explore Psalm 34. These words are the lyrics of "Psalm 34," recorded by the Brooklyn Tabernacle Choir. In verses 4-5, what does David tell us about seeking God?

_____

_____

_____

What does he say about God in verses 6-7?

_____

_____

_____

What does David call us to do in verses 8-9?

_____

_____

_____

In verse 10, what is a benefit of seeking the Lord?

_____

_____

_____

What lessons does David want to teach us in verses 11-14?

_____

_____

_____

What is one of your favorite praise and worship songs? How do the melody and lyrics impact you?

_____

_____

_____

Although we don't have much information about the details of our life in heaven, I believe it will look a lot like musical theater. We will sing praises to God continually, overcome by being fully in His presence, unable to stop our voices from singing songs of worship and adoration. In fact, what does Paul tell us to do in Ephesians 5:19?

_____

_____

_____

Let's join with David and live each day with a song in our heart, praising our King and enjoying the benefits that music brings to our souls. Use music today in your exercise routine to focus on God as you love Him with all your strength.

I will praise You at all times, Lord, and Your praise will continually be in my mouth. I glorify You and exalt Your Name, singing songs of worship and adulation to the King of my heart. Amen.

—— DAY 3: LAMENT

When my heart is overwhelmed, I cry out to You, O Lord. Lead me to the Rock that is higher than I, for You have been a shelter for me.

What do you do when you encounter a problem? Especially a problem that seems unsolvable? One thing you likely do is cry out to God. This pleading to God for help is known in the psalms as a "lament." These types of psalms make up about one-third of the book. There are many reasons David or another author may have written a lament, or complaint, poem. It could have been due to personal danger, national crises, or general injustice. But whatever the cause, the poem was spoken directly to God and asked Him to intervene and correct the situation and deal with the people who caused the problem.

An example of a lament psalm written by David is Psalm 5. Let's analyze his words and discover how he prayed to God when faced with difficulties. How did he begin the poem in verses 1-2?

_____

_____

_____

What did David do each morning (verse 3)?

_____

_____

_____

Verses 4-6 give us a hint as to the reason for David's complaint. Whom did he talk about in these verses?

_____

_____

_____

In verse 7 David paused his complaint. What did he talk about in this verse?

_____

_____

_____

What did David ask God to do to his enemies in verses 8-10?

_____

_____

_____

What reason did he give in verse 10 for his request?

_____

_____

_____

The psalm ends with verses 11-12? How are these verses different from the previous three verses.

_____

_____

_____

Psalm 5 follows a pattern that is found in most lament psalms.[6] Identify the verses from Psalm 5 that go with each of these three parts of the lament.

Beginning: The problem or disaster _____

Middle: The psalmist's request from God _____

End: Resolution or hope of a resolution _____

Psalm 5 differs slightly from this pattern because there is a bit of hope in the center of the psalm. Verse 7 reads, "But I, by your great love, can come into your house; in reverence I bow down toward your holy temple." What do you think David meant by writing these verses in the midst of his complaint?

_____

_____

_____

Read Psalm 13 and identify the three parts of the lament prayer in this psalm.

Beginning: The problem or disaster _____

Middle: The psalmist's request from God _____

End: Resolution or hope of a resolution _____

You may notice that these lament psalms end on a positive note. The writers knew they faced calamities outside their control. They cried out to God for help. But they also knew the greatness and supremacy of their God. They depended on Him for all they needed. Even when they faltered, they knew He would be faithful to them. It has been said that we should not tell God how big our problems are but tell our problems how big our God is!

Living a consistently healthy life may be an overwhelming task for you. You may cry out to God for help in food and exercise choices, and He is waiting eagerly to hear from you, ready to empower you to put Him first. You can depend on Him; He is faithful forever. Tell Him now whatever is on your heart and ask for His unending power to win the victory over temptations and testing.

_____

_____

_____

I trust in Your unfailing love, my Father, and my heart rejoices in Your salvation. I will sing the Lord's praise, for He has been and continues to be good to me! Amen.

—— DAY 4: PETITION AND PENITENCE

Lord, do not forsake me; do not be far from me, my God. Come quickly to help me, my Lord and my Savior.

Disney movies often cast a princess or female lead in a situation where she has a great desire to be fulfilled. This results in her singing an "I want" song. Snow White sings "I'm Wishing" about the man she wants to meet and fall in love with. Ariel sings about becoming "Part of Your World" and wishes for legs in *The Little Mermaid*. In *Frozen* Elsa sings "Let It Go," expressing her desire to be herself and not hide her powers. Perhaps the largest percentage of our prayers involve our "I wants": our petitions telling God what we want, whether for ourselves or someone else.

David's songs included petition, which is often part of psalms of lament. Read Psalm 40:11-17. We do not know the circumstances behind this psalm, but David had many instances in his life when he would have petitioned God in this way. Verse 12 only says, "For troubles without number surround me; my sins have overtaken me, and I cannot see. They are more than the hairs of my head, and my heart fails within me." As you read verses 11 and 13-17, identify what David requests from God in each one.

Verse 11 _____

Verse 13 _____

Verse 14 _____

Verse 15 _____

Verse 16 _____

Verse 17 _____

We can see in this prayer David's deep despair and longing for God's intervention to relieve his pain. He was not too proud to ask God for help, and he honestly told God what he needed. Recall a time you prayed to God, asking for His help and deliverance. What was the prayer and the outcome?

_____

_____

_____

Another type of psalm is that of penitence. David expressed sorrow over his sin in several songs, including Psalm 38. "Psalm 38 is the prayer of an individual suffering from an illness that he views as a punishment inflicted by God. The psalmist confesses his sins and asks God for forgiveness."[7] Read this psalm. How did David begin this psalm in verse 1?

_____

_____

_____

How had David's sin affected him (verses 2-4)?

_____

_____

_____

What physical ailments did David believe he suffered due to his sin (verses 5-8)?

_____

_____

_____

In verse 9, David expressed his transparency before God. "All my longings lie open before you, Lord; my sighing is not hidden from you." In verses 10-14, what are some of the conditions David listed that resulted from his sin?

_____

_____

_____

What did David say in verse 18?

_____

_____

_____

How did he end the prayer in verses 20-21?

_____

_____

_____

One theme of this psalm is the devastating effects of sin on our lives. Unconfessed sin and chronic unhealthy behavior can hurt us in all four parts of our being. God expects us to take care of our bodies as His temple (1 Corinthians 6:19-20), and when we don't, we may suffer physically. Hiding our sin from God only causes internal pain and stress. Thankfully the Holy Spirit works in us to reveal our sin and help us recover. The only remedy is confession and repentance: agreeing with God that what we are doing is wrong and seeking His help to change our behaviors. Is there any sin in your life today? Do you need to confess any sin to God and ask for His forgiveness and help for repentance? Are there any behaviors that can cause you pain?

_____

_____

_____

We will look at another of David's psalms of penitence in Week 6. In this psalm he did not hide his sin from God and trusted God's faithfulness to forgive Him when he confessed and repented of his sin. When we sin, we too can depend on God to forgive and heal us. Read 1 John 1:9, or recite it from memory if you can, and record it here.

_____

_____

_____

The heart of this king sometimes suffered from hurt, despair, and brokenness. The words of his songs resonate with us because we also cry out to God with our petitions and penitence. God is ready and eager to hear our prayers and answer them with His deliverance and forgiveness. All we need do is turn to Him in humility and honesty with faith.

Lord, I wait for You; You will answer, Lord my God. I'm thankful I can bring my petitions and my prayers of penitence to You, and that You faithfully hear and answer my prayers. Free me from sinful behaviors that hurt me and bring dishonor to You. Amen.

—— DAY 5: CELEBRATION AND THANKSGIVING

Many, Lord my God, are the wonders you have done, the things you planned for us. None can compare with you; were I to speak and tell of your deeds, they would be too many to declare.

A little bird suffered greatly, lacking food, shelter, and feathers. He constantly complained about his plight. One day he cried out to God and asked how long his suffering would last. God answered that he would have seven years until his difficulties would end. God also told the bird to say, "Thank You, God, for everything." The little bird started using these words when faced with difficult situations. When he was hungry, he said, "Thank You, God, for everything." When he was hot under the blazing sun, he said, "Thank You, God, for everything." When he saw other birds living life without his problems, he said, "Thank You, God, for everything." Soon the little bird was happy even in the midst of his anguish. He found a pond of water and a tree to provide shelter. He began to grow feathers and get stronger. A week passed and the little bird asked God why he was now happy when he had been told his misery would last seven years. God told the little bird that He had collapsed his seven-year forecast into seven days. "The power of gratitude can change long hours of waiting to mere minutes. It is more powerful than any situation."[8]

David wrote thanks to God in his psalms, often celebrating Who God is in his songs. Yesterday we looked at the second half of Psalm 40, and today we'll revisit this song and explore the first part. Read Psalm 40:1-5. For what did David praise God in verses 2-3?

_____

_____

_____

Notice verse 1: "I waited patiently for the Lord; he turned to me and heard my cry." David gave us a little backstory here. At some time in the past he asked God for help

73

but had to wait to receive the answer. Now he was thanking God for what He had done. In verse 3 what resulted from God's answer to his prayer?

_____

_____

_____

How is the "one who trusts in the Lord" blessed (verse 4)?

_____

_____

_____

What did David say about God in verse 5?

_____

_____

_____

The second part of Psalm 40 is filled with petition and lament. Why do you suppose David started this psalm with celebration and thanksgiving?

_____

_____

_____

Look up Psalm 124. Why was David thankful (verses 1-5)?

_____

_____

_____

How does he end the psalm in verse 8?

_____

_____

_____

Finally read Psalm 133:1-3. How does David celebrate God in verses 1-2?

_____

_____

_____

In verse 2 to what does David compare the cause of his thankfulness?

_____

_____

_____

Take a moment to consider the content of your prayers to God. How often do you thank Him and celebrate the victories He brings?

_____

_____

_____

What has God done in your life recently for which you can thank Him?

_____

_____

_____

David, the man after God's own heart and fit to be king, thanked God regularly, even during difficult circumstances. Write a prayer to God thanking Him for blessings in your life. Celebrate the God of all creation Who loves and cares for you.

_____

_____

_____

Thank You, gracious Father, for all You have done for me. You have saved me and given me purpose. You protect me and provide for me. You speak to me through Your Word and help me learn to obey You. Great are You, Lord, and mighty is Your Name. Amen.

—— DAY 6: REFLECTION AND APPLICATION

Your Word is precious to me, O Lord. It feeds me with truth and hope. It guides me in Your right paths. It fills me with Your love. Speak to me now, Holy Father.

David's songs recorded in the book of Psalms provide encouragement and wisdom for us today. Some of these poems follow a pattern such as we saw in Psalm 40. Part of the psalm expresses David's pain and concern, while another part is full of praise and thanksgiving. It resembles a journal entry that pours despair out of the heart but fills it up again with hope from God.

Author, speaker, and podcaster Carlos Whittaker shared his story of struggling with anxiety. His condition improved through therapy and other tools but he wasn't completely healed. He reflected on his prayers and found that they were full of problems. He was feeding his anxiety by focusing on his complaints. He looked at the prayers of Jesus in the gospels and noticed that He often did not only pray the problem. He prayed the promise instead. So Carlos changed the way he prayed, using scripture that applied to the problem. Instead of praying, "God, I'm so depressed; I'll never get out of this," he prayed, "I will fear no evil, for Thou art with me. Satan has no power over me. Greater is He who is in me than he who is in the world. No weapon formed against me shall stand." Carlos said the more you are in the Word, the more the Word is in you and the more the Word comes out of you in prayer. His anxiety decreased dramatically once he began to pray the promise instead of the problem. After learning and practicing this truth, his teenage daughter was hospitalized with a serious, unknown condition. In this traumatic situation he experienced peace and hope. She eventually received a diagnosis and successful treatment. But the miracle for Carlos was his victory over anxiety by praying God's promises instead of his problems.[9]

We can see this practice in David's prayers too. He often started a psalm with pain and protests but ended with praise and thanks to God. David based his confidence in God because he knew His character. He walked with God in the past and experienced His protection and provision. He believed God would continue to take care of him no matter what happened.

Let's practice this model for prayer from David's songs. As you respond in the blanks below, consider including scripture where you can. First, tell God what is on your heart, your deepest desires and longings.

_____

_____

_____

Next, recount how God has helped you in the past.

_____

_____

_____

Finally, end your prayer with praise and thanksgiving to God.

When we fill our entire being—heart, soul, mind, and body—with the promises of God, our problems shrink in comparison to His mighty power. Here's an example of praying the promise rather than the problem. Notice that the problems are still within the prayer but they are surrounded by God's Word and faith in Him.

Holy Father, I thank You that any temptation to make an unhealthy choice today also comes with a way of escape from you. I know that You are with me in every step I take at my job and with my family and friends. Your strength supports me when I'm on the road and Your riches in Christ Jesus meet all my needs when I struggle financially. When I face deep waters of physical agony, You are with me and will not allow the pains to overwhelm me. When others make choices that hurt me, You are my hiding place. I claim Your victory over sin, Lord, for You have made me more than a conqueror through Jesus Christ my Lord. I am walking in Your paths of righteous for Your Name's sake. My eyes are fixed on Jesus, the author and finisher of my faith, the beginning and the end, and the soon-coming triumphant King. You are my all in all, and I love You. Amen.

(This prayer incorporates these scripture verses: 1 Corinthians 10:13, Deuteronomy 31:6, Philippians 4:13 and 19, Isaiah 43:2, Psalm 91, Romans 8:37, Psalm 23:3, Hebrews 12:2, and Revelation 22:12-13.)

Thank You, God, that Your Word accomplishes what You desire and never returns to You empty. As I include Your promises in my prayers to focus on Your sufficiency rather than my inadequacy, increase my faith in You, my loving Lord Who is compassionate, gracious, slow to anger, and full of loyal love and faithfulness. I love You, Father. Amen.

—— DAY 7: REFLECTION AND APPLICATION
Your song of hope and love fills my heart with peace and strength. I worship You, almighty God, my Lord and King. Show me Your face as I seek You now.

Write this week's memory verses here.

During this week's study, you have had opportunities to investigate the lyrics of David's songs. Use the content and processes in today's reflection. Below are some prompts for your meditation and journaling.

- **Create a soundtrack of your life** or for a specific season of your life. List the names of songs that represent your experiences and resonate with you. You can use an app to create a playlist of the songs that represent you and use them in your exercise routine or any time. How do these songs impact you?
- **Choose a psalm and find or create images to illustrate it.** For example, Psalm 121 mentions mountains, shade, sun (day), and moon (night).
- **"The Book of Psalms** is divided into five parts, parallel to the Five Books of Moses (Genesis through Deuteronomy). It is further subdivided into seven parts, one for each day in the week, and further divided into 30 divisions, for each day of the month."[10] Psalms was created as a daily prayer book for the Israelites, as reflected in the book's first two chapters. Schedule time each day to read one of the chapters in the book of Psalms, starting at chapter 1 and reading through chapter 150. Reading the entire book in this way will take about five months. Use the words as daily meditation on God and His character. Note how the types of psalms progress from chapters 1-150. You may notice there are more psalms of praise as you go from the beginning to the end. Record any thoughts you have in your journal.
- **Find a song that encourages you** in this process. You may document the lyrics and record your own reflections on them, or you could illustrate them with sketches or images you locate. Several examples of songs were referenced in the Day 2 lesson. They include "Whom Shall I Fear (God of Angel Armies)" by Chris Tomlin (2012), "My Soul Will Wait (Psalm 62)" by Sovereign Grace (2022), and "Psalm 34" by the Brooklyn Tabernacle Choir (2018). Another one is Chris Tomlin's "Forever" (2001), based on Psalm 13.

Your journal holds a very private and personal process; therefore, share it carefully. If social media is a healthy place for you, use these hashtags for posting your words, images, other reflections, or personal stories from this study: #fp4h and #fp4hfitforaking. You can view my journal and others' entries using these hashtags.

I sing a song of praise for my God and King. For He found me and redeemed me from my sin and despair. I praise Him with my whole being as I sing joyful songs to Him every day. May the music of my heart spill over into my walk, leading me to love God and others for His Name's sake. Amen.

1 Jeffrey Kranz, "The 8 Types of Psalms in the Bible," Overview Bible (2014), https://overviewbible.com/kinds-of-psalms/.

2 "Great Lessons King David Teaches about Worship," Afro Gist Media, https://afrogistmedia.com/5-great-lessons-king-david-teaches-about-worship.

3 Jeffery Kranz, "The 8 Types of Psalms in the Bible," "Overview Bible" (2014), https://overviewbible.com/kinds-of-psalms/.

4 Honor Whiteman, "The Power of Music: How It Can Benefit Health," Medical News Today (2015), https://www.medicalnewstoday.com/articles/302903#Reducing-pain-and-anxiety.

5 Camilla Klein, "Discover the Surprising Number of Christian Worship Songs from David's Psalms," Christian Educators Academy (2023), https://christianeducatorsacademy.com/discover-the-surprising-number-of-christian-worship-songs-from-davids-psalms/.

6 Harry Hagan, "Laments: The Prayer Psalms or Psalms of Petition," Elements of Biblical Poetry, Palni Press, https://pressbooks.palni.org/elementsofbiblicalpoetry/chapter/13-laments/.

7 "What are the penitential psalms?" Got Questions, https://www.gotquestions.org/penitential-psalms.html.

8 "Story: Thank You God for Everything," Prayables (2020), https://prayables.com/story-thank-you-god-for-everything-012118/.

9 "Carlos Whitaker on Praying the Promise instead of the Problem," The Alli Worthington Show, June 22, 2020.

10 "King David and the Psalms," Chabad.org, https://www.chabad.org/library/article_cdo/aid/2050/jewish/King-David-and-the-Psalms.htm.

WEEK FIVE: DAVID'S INTEGRITY

SCRIPTURE MEMORY VERSE

Who may ascend the mountain of the LORD? Who may stand in his holy place? The one who has clean hands and a pure heart, who does not trust in an idol or swear by a false god. Psalm 24:3-4

The day finally arrived. David became Israel's king after Saul's death in battle and seven years of waiting for all the tribes of Israel to crown him. He was ready to fulfill God's calling to lead His people. What plans did David have for his reign? We may have a glimpse into his thoughts in Psalm 101. One source writes, "He had but recently ascended the throne. The abuses and confusions of Saul's last troubled years had to be reformed. The new king felt that he was God's viceroy; and here declares what he will strive to make his monarchy—a copy of God's."[1] In verse 2 David says, "I will walk with *integrity* of heart within my house" (ESV). His greatest concern was not about self-aggrandizement, revenge on his enemies, wealth, or fame. Instead, he writes, "I will sing of steadfast love and justice; to you, O LORD, I will make music. I will ponder the way that is blameless" (Psalm 101:1-2a, ESV). He focused on the One Who called him when he was a young unknown shepherd, and he committed to following Him with his entire heart, soul, mind, and strength.

On the idea of integrity, David Guzek writes,

> In the Old Testament, the Hebrew word translated "integrity" means "the condition of being without blemish, completeness, perfection, sincerity, soundness, uprightness, wholeness." Integrity in the New Testament means "honesty and adherence to a pattern of good works."[2]

It has been said that integrity is who you are and what you do when no one is looking. For those of us working on fitness goals through First Place for Health, that might involve honestly recording our food intake on our trackers. It includes consistently developing the healthy habits taught in our program, like regular exercise and balanced food choices. And walking in integrity consists of putting God first in everything we do and doing it to honor Him, not ourselves.

Last week for *Fit for a King* we learned about David's songs recorded in Psalms.

- David praised God in song, applauding Him for His character and His actions.
- Enjoying music has benefits, and David's psalms have inspired numerous hymns and modern Christian songs.
- Many of David's songs were laments, crying out to God for help, expressing his deepest emotions in poetry.
- Petition was included in David's songs, asking God for help for himself and others, as well as penitence, begging God's forgiveness when he sinned.
- Thankfulness and celebration were part of David's songs, even when he was in the midst of trouble.

During this week's study we will examine David's integrity. How did his initial commitment to walk the blameless path play out during his reign? And what can we learn about integrity from his life? As we encounter God through His Word, we have opportunities to examine our own walk with Him and evaluate our own integrity as committed followers of Christ.

—— DAY 1: INTEGRITY WITH LEADERS

Holy Father, how I love and adore You. My life belongs to You, and I desire to know You more intimately. Show me Yourself through Your Word as I enter into Your presence now.

Complete the blanks below to practice learning this week's memory verses.

Who may _____ the _____ of the Lord? Who may _____ in his _____ place? The one who has _____ hands and a _____ heart, who does not trust in an _____ or swear by a false _____.

_____ _____ : _____

In these verses David is describing aspects of integrity. What four prerequisites does he list for one who seeks God (verse 4)?

_____

_____

_____

How did David live up to this description? Let's look first at how David lived with integrity in relationship to those in authority over him. After David slayed Goliath, he won many military victories, earning him accolades and prestige. This praise caused Saul to be jealous of David, and he began to look for ways he could eliminate him. Read 1 Samuel 18:17. What did Saul offer David and why?

_____

_____

_____

How did David respond in verse 18?

_____

_____

_____

King Saul's first daughter was given to another man to marry. But Saul learned that another daughter, Michal, was in love with David. He thought he could use the situation to his advantage (1 Samuel 18:20). He had his attendants talk to David; what did they say to him (verses 22-23)?

_____

_____

_____

How did David respond in verse 23?

_____

_____

_____

How did David show integrity in this situation?

_____

_____

_____

Saul hatched a plan, hoping to get David killed in battle. What was this plan (verse 25)?

_____

_____

_____

David accepted Saul's challenge. What was the result (verse 27)?

_____

_____

_____

Although Saul planned to harm him, David served him faithfully. God protected him in battle, and he was successful. On another occasion, Saul hunted David down in order to kill him. Saul went into a cave alone, unaware that David and his men were in the back of the cave. What did David's men encourage him to do (1 Samuel 24:4)?

_____

_____

_____

David didn't kill Saul but did cut off a corner of the king's robe while Saul was unaware of his presence. He immediately regretted what he had done and told his men not to harm Saul (verses 5-7). How did David refer to Saul in verse 6?

_____

_____

_____

After Saul left the cave and rejoined his men, David called out to him and prostrated himself before him (verse 10). Read verse 11 and summarize David's statement to Saul.

_____

_____

_____

Saul stopped his pursuit of David for a time. But a similar situation is recorded in 1 Samuel 26. David had another opportunity to kill Saul in his sleep, but he refused to take advantage of him. Finally, let's revisit David's eulogy for Saul and Jonathan. What did he say about King Saul after his death in 2 Samuel 1:26?

_____

_____

_____

His words of praise seem strange considering how Saul treated him. He had been in danger for his life for years because Saul chased him and tried to kill him. But David never forgot that Saul was the anointed king of Israel, and he consistently treated him with the respect his position commanded, no matter how Saul abused him. David ensured that Saul and Jonathan had a proper burial (2 Samuel 21:10-14). Even after Saul's death, David acted with integrity toward his predecessor. This behavior is not the norm, both then and now.

What can we learn about integrity from David's respect for authority? How do we treat the authorities in our lives? Our bosses? Leaders of organizations to which we belong? Government officials? What do you think David's integrity means in our own relationship to authorities in our lives?

_____

_____

_____

What does Romans 13:1-5 say about how we should respond to authorities?

_____

_____

_____

David proved himself a man of integrity before God put him on Israel's throne. He was faithful in small things, so God trusted his integrity for bigger things. He obeyed authorities as if he was obeying God, and he did it with true deference, not gritting his teeth with resentment. His attitude toward authorities showed his attitude toward God.

God has called us to honor Him with our bodies through healthy habits. How does our response to this call reflect our attitude toward God's authority in our lives?

_____

_____

_____

Father, I thank You for Your authority in my life. You always want what's best for me, and I trust You as my Lord and King. Develop in me a heart of submission to you and other authorities in my life, always reflecting my devotion to You. Amen.

—— DAY 2: INTEGRITY WITH POSITION

My gracious and loving Father, I come to You with all my concerns and celebrations. How grateful I am that I can talk to You about anything and that You always hear me. Let Your Word speak to my heart in these moments together.

David was not immediately crowned Israel's king after Saul's death. The custom of the time was that a relative of the king would ascend to the throne. David continued to act with integrity as the politics of the day played out, waiting for God to act rather than taking action himself. Turn to 2 Samuel 2:3-4. Where did David and his community settle and what happened there?

_____

_____

_____

How long did David serve as king in Hebron over Judah (verse 11)?

_____

In the meantime the head of King Saul's army, Abner, took one of the king's sons, Ish-Bosheth, and led the people in anointing him king in Saul's place over the other tribes of Israel. David did not lead his army against Ish-Bosheth. He waited for God to accomplish His calling in his life, knowing He would do what He promised. How do David's actions demonstrate his integrity?

_____

_____

_____

However, Joab, the leader of David's army did fight against Abner and his followers. Eventually, Abner came to David's side after falling out with Ish-Bosheth. Read 2 Samuel 3:17-18. What did Abner tell the leaders of Israel?

_____

_____

_____

Joab killed Abner in revenge for Abner killing his brother Asahel. David mourned Abner's death and reprimanded Joab for his murder (2 Samuel 3:31-35). How did the people respond to David's actions (verses 35-36)?

_____

_____

_____

David's restraint from forcing himself into the king's position proved to be beneficial to his relationship to the people he ruled. They saw he was not power-hungry but patient and devoted to God. This integrity served him and his people well for most of David's life. He was finally crowned king over all the tribes of Israel and made Jerusalem his capital. One thing that most new kings did at that time was kill all the relatives of the previous king. That prevented anyone from the former king's family opposing the new king and trying to dethrone him. But David did not follow this pattern of violence. After becoming firmly established as king, what question did he ask in 2 Samuel 9:1?

He discovered Jonathan had a surviving son, Mephibosheth. What does 2 Samuel 4:4 say about Mephibosheth?

Put yourself in Mephibosheth's place. He grieved over his grandfather and father who were killed in battle. His uncle Ish-Bosheth had been murdered. He knew a new king was on the throne. He knew the practice of the day: the new king killed the former king's family. David's men arrived at his home to take him to the king. Surely he must have been terrified, thinking his end was near. Find 2 Samuel 9:6. What did he do when he came into the king's presence?

What did King David say to Mephibosheth in verse 7?

Why did David want to care for Mephibosheth? He had made a covenant with Jonathan years ago, and in this covenant they both promised to care for each other's families as if they were their own. David acted with integrity in keeping his covenant with Jonathan, even if no one else knew of their agreement. He kept his promise to his friend, and Mephibosheth, lame and alone, became his adopted son.

Asaph was a leader of worship during David's reign. What did he say about David's rule over his people in Psalm 78:72?

_____

_____

_____

David did not use his position to benefit himself but continually practiced integrity, showing his concern to do what God led him to do and not carry out his own agenda. In your own life how can you practice integrity as modeled by David?

_____

_____

_____

Father, you have put me in this place at this time for Your purposes. You have put others in authority over me and You have given me authority over others. Help me to follow Your Spirit's leadership in my heart so that I act with integrity in all I do, so others will know I belong to You. Amen.

—— DAY 3: INTEGRITY DURING CRISIS

We live in a fallen, broken world, Lord. How it must hurt Your heart to see Your perfect creation damaged and full of rebellion. Equip me to live with integrity in a world that rejects You.

In order to avoid the constant threat of death by King Saul, David, his troops, and all their families escaped to the land of the Philistines. For over a year they lived in Ziklag. In 1 Samuel 30, David and his men returned to their home base after going to battle. What did they find upon their arrival (verse 3)?

_____

_____

_____

Imagine the horror these men faced: everything they held dear captured or destroyed. What does verse 5 tell us about David's situation in this disaster?

_____

_____

_____

His family and his home were gone. "But David found strength in the Lord his God" (1 Samuel 30:6). When things were as bad as they might get, David continued to put his faith in Yahweh. How did David respond to this tragedy and what did God tell him to do (verses 7-8)?

_____

_____

_____

David took some of his troops to rescue their people and possessions. Some of the men were exhausted and couldn't go on, so they stayed behind and guarded their supplies. What was the result of David's attack on those who had plundered their community (verse 18-20)?

_____

_____

_____

When David and the troops who were with him returned to the men who had guarded their supplies, there was an argument. Those who fought didn't believe that the plunder they had collected from their enemies should be shared with those who had stayed behind (verse 22). Read verses 23-25. What was David's response to this conflict?

_____

_____

_____

David demonstrated integrity and leadership in a time of crisis. He lost his own home and wives in this raid, and he led his men with wisdom and honor. Due to his dependence on God, they rescued their families and possessions. He made it clear that his men were a team and no matter what part they played in the mission, they all deserved to share in the rewards. In fact, David went on to share the enemy's plunder with other people who had supported him during his time of running from Saul. Read verse 26 and record David's actions.

_____

_____

_____

Our world calls us to be selfish and do what benefits us most with no regard to how our actions affect others. It was the same in David's world. Leaders didn't share or give away the loot they captured in battle. Kings were oppressive and violent, ruling by fear and force. But David saw his men as equals before God and treated them all with dignity and compassion. He was generous and remembered those who had been good to him. Even in a time of crisis he didn't abandon his integrity. He went to God for wisdom and obeyed His Word.

Tennis great Andy Roddick was poised to win. In the second game of the 16th round of the 2005 Italia Masters he had triple match point, three chances to defeat his opponent Fernando Verdasco. He was the top seed in this tournament and now had a chance to move to the next round of play. After faulting on his first serve, Verdasco served the ball for a second time, attempting an ace. However, the linesman called the ball out, awarding the point to Roddick. As Verdasco came to the net to congratulate Roddick on winning the match, Roddick stood looking at the place where the ball had landed. He faced a crisis: he knew the ball was in although it had been called out. He went to the umpire and told him that the ball had been in. He showed the umpire the place on the line where the ball had landed and left a mark on the clay surface. The umpire changed the ruling and awarded the point to Verdasco, who amazingly came back from the apparent loss and won the game, the set, and finally the match. Roddick's honesty cost him money, prestige, and victory in the highly competitive world of tennis. But he didn't seem to think his actions were unusual. "Maybe I should have stood on the mark," Roddick joked with reporters. "I don't think I did anything extraordinary, the umpire would have come down and said the same too. I just saved him the trip."[3] Roddick is remembered more for this act of integrity than he would have been had he won the tournament.

Our integrity stands out in stark contrast in a world focused on pride and self-centeredness. Following Christ means living by a higher standard knowing everything we do represents our King to people who don't know His amazing love. When we encounter a crisis, it is tempting to take the easy way and sacrifice our integrity. Have you faced a time where chose integrity over selfishness? What was the situation and how did you respond?

_____

_____

_____

I am challenged daily to follow You and live with integrity because the world system is in opposition to You, Father. It is easy to compromise and do what I think is best. Help me to trust in You rather than my own understanding, acknowledging You in all my ways as You direct my paths. Amen.

—— DAY 4: INTEGRITY WITH RESOURCES

Every good and perfect gift I have comes from You, Father of light in Whom there is no shifting shadows of change. I surrender my all to You now as I open Your Word.

King David ruled Israel well for decades. One aspect of ruling is managing resources with integrity, and he did this well. One story that reflects his financial responsibility concerns the purchase of a threshing floor, which was a level outdoor area used for threshing sheaves of grain—often located on the top of a rock or hilltop. Turn to 2 Samuel 24:18-25. The setting for this passage involves a plague that threatened Israel that David had caused through a rebellious act. We will look at the cause of the plague in next week's lessons, but here we see how David handled his mistake, a true test of integrity. In verses 18-19 what direction from God did David receive through the prophet Gad?

_____

_____

_____

How did Araunah, the owner of the threshing floor, respond to King David's mission in verses 22-23?

_____

_____

_____

It was certainly in the king's power to take the threshing floor without any payment at all. But what did David say to Araunah in verse 24?

_____

_____

_____

His integrity is especially outstanding when compared to King Ahab, a future king of the Northern Kingdom of Israel. Look up 1 Kings 21:2. What did King Ahab say to Naboth?

_____

_____

_____

How did Naboth respond in verse 3?

_____

_____

_____

Although King Ahab offered a fair price for the land, Naboth knew his land was bound up in his family's legacy and didn't want to jeopardize his children's inheritance. How did King Ahab respond to Naboth's refusal (verse 4)?

_____

_____

_____

Can you imagine a more immature way to react? King Ahab pouted and when his wife Queen Jezebel found out what happened, she had Naboth killed and took the land for her husband. Their ruthless selfishness was called out by the prophet Elijah who predicted their violent deaths. King Ahab was greedy and did not act with integrity. He was not fit to be a king. However, David showed great integrity in his dealings with Araunah.

Read David's words in Psalm 62:10. What warning does he offer?

_____

_____

_____

What does the author of Psalm 128:1-2 tell us about our attitude toward our resources?

_____

_____

_____

What does Jesus say about our attitude toward what we own in Matthew 6:19-21?

What is your attitude toward your possessions?

When a Christian leader is accused of mishandling ministry money, the world is quick to attack him, discrediting the name of Jesus and His church. People who are fit for a king know that none of their resources truly belongs to them. They are all on loan from God. We are called to be good stewards of what He has entrusted to us. That includes our time and talents, our choices about food and exercise, and our relationships with others. The measure of our love for God is sometimes best revealed in how we use the resources at our disposal. Let's walk with integrity as we use what God has given us for His kingdom and His glory.

I surrender my resources to You, Father, knowing that I have nothing without You. I am incredibly blessed with earthly possessions but they are meaningless apart from You. Help me to walk with integrity as I make decisions about how to use money and other assets according to Your will. Amen.

—— DAY 5: INTEGRITY TO THE END

You have plans for me, my God, and I want to walk faithfully in them today. Show me Your wisdom and Your power during my quiet time with You so I may know Your truth and Your heart.

Dr. Allen V. Astin was the director of the United States' National Institute for Standards and Technology (NIST) in the 1950s and 1960s. During his tenure a battery additive was tested and shown to be ineffective in prolonging battery life. Under intense pressure to have the additive verified as successful, it was tested again—with the same results. MIT had opposing reports about the product's viability, and the manufacturer and Congress conducted intense investigations into the NIST. Astin continued to support the testing protocols and results but political pressure forced him to resign. Later it was confirmed that the NIST was right and Dr. Astin was reinstated. His leadership during this time of crisis confirmed the government agency's integrity and stature in the science community. When he died, the eulogy for Dr. Astin included this story of strength under fire. His two children, John Astin (actor and director and professor at John Hopkins University's Theater Department) and Alexander (Sandy) Astin (Founding Director of the Higher Education Research Institute at UCLA) carried on his legacy of excellence in their respective fields.[4]

David exemplified integrity to the end of his life and passed on that example to his nation and family as well. As we saw in 2 Samuel 7 David wanted to build a temple for God, and God said his son would build it instead. The desire for the temple never left David's mind, however. He could have left the project entirely in Solomon's hands. But his integrity kept him focused on carrying out whatever was needed to ensure the temple's construction became a reality after he was gone. Once he became ruler over all Israel, David continued to fight battles as he established his kingdom. 2 Samuel 8 lists several nations he defeated. What does verse 6 say about the source of David's victories?

_____

_____

_____

What did David do with the spoils from his battles and the tributes that the conquered nations paid to him (verses 11-12)?

_____

_____

_____

Dedicating these items to God meant they were to be used for His purposes, not for David or the nation's wealth. Read 1 Chronicles 22:5. Toward the end of his life, what did David do and why?

_____

_____

_____

Verses 1-4 details some of the things David bought with his enemies' wealth. What are some of them?

_____

_____

_____

What did David tell Solomon about the supplies he collected for the temple's construction in verse 14?

But the preparation for the temple project was not the only thing that David left for his son Solomon, the next king of Israel. Find 1 Kings 9:4-5, part of a conversation God had with Solomon after David's death. What did God promise Solomon He would do for him in verse 5?

What was Solomon's part in this agreement (verse 4)?

God encouraged Solomon to follow the model David set for him and the entire nation: "walk before me faithfully with integrity of heart and uprightness" (1 Kings 9:4). The Hebrew phrase "integrity of heart" carries with it the idea of a heart that is undivided and completely devoted to God. David's inner being was so loyal to God that he could not help but act with integrity, and his son Solomon was called to do the same as the new king of Israel. How does David reflect on this idea in Psalm 86:11?

How does Mark 12:30, the foundational verse of First Place for Health, also reflect this idea?

What does living with an undivided heart look like for you?

_____

_____

_____

As we consider leading a life marked by integrity, let us dedicate ourselves to following God with an undivided heart, completely devoted to Him for our entire lives. And may we leave an example of integrity to those we leave behind.

Father God, I want to live my life so that it reflects Your love for me. I desire to consistently walk in Your truths with an undivided heart, completely devoted to You. Show me today where I can leave a mark of integrity with my words and actions. Amen.

—— DAY 6: REFLECTION AND APPLICATION

Thank You for this day, my God. You have a purpose for me to fulfill and You have given me everything I need according to Your riches in glory in Christ Jesus. Use this quiet time alone with You to focus me on that purpose.

Write this week's memory verses here.

_____

_____

_____

Another biblical figure who exemplifies integrity is Daniel. Let's look at three examples of integrity in his life. The first is in Daniel 1:8. When presented with the opportunity to eat sumptuously from the king's table and break Mosaic laws, how did Daniel respond?

_____

_____

_____

In Daniel 4 he received an interpretation of a dream that King Nebuchadnezzar wanted explained. It contained really bad news and Daniel could have lied. Telling a king news like that could get a prophet killed. Read Daniel 4:19-27. What did he do?

_____

_____

_____

Finally, in Daniel's most famous story in the Bible, he was thrown into the lion's den and survived. The reason he found himself there was due to his integrity. Other officials were jealous of Daniel's position as second only to the king. What does Daniel 6:4 say that they tried to do?

_____

_____

_____

What obstacles did they face in discrediting Daniel?

_____

_____

_____

What does verse 5 mean?

_____

_____

_____

Daniel Taylor discusses integrity in *Letters to my Children*:

> He writes that integrity "means wholeness, unity." When we sin, we become divided and less whole. Each time that happens, we become less of who God intends us to be. God desires that we worship only him, with all of our lives. So often we can hide an idol from the public, but in worshipping it secretly we become less human and less of who God intends us to be."[5]

The world calls us to live for ourselves, but God calls us to live for Him. As you meditate today on the life of Daniel consider these questions.

How do you reflect integrity in your food choices?

_____

_____

_____

How do you reflect integrity with speaking the truth in love?

_____

_____

_____

How do you reflect integrity in your work?

_____

_____

_____

As you finish your quiet time with God in prayer, meditate on Titus 2:7-8.

> In everything set... an example by doing what is good. In your teaching show integrity, seriousness and soundness of speech that cannot be condemned, so that those who oppose you may be ashamed because they have nothing bad to say about us.

Thank You for Daniel's life of integrity that is recorded in Your Word. Only through Your power and the Holy Spirit's direction can I embody his example. I trust You today to help me make the best choices with food, exercise, time, and talents. Amen.

—— DAY 7: REFLECTION AND APPLICATION

You, Lord, are righteous and inscrutable, abounding in love to all who call on You. I lay all my cares and pains before You now so that I may worship and adore You with my entire being.

This week we have considered the integrity David epitomized in his lifetime. As we reflect on these examples of uprightness, let's find applications to our own lives. Here are some prompts for meditation and/or journaling.

- **Draw or locate an image of a medal,** preferably a service medal like the Medal of Honor. Above the image write "Medal of Integrity." Below the image make a list of the qualifications one would need to receive the medal. Use scripture verses where appropriate.
- **Think about someone you know or have known who you believe best exemplifies integrity.** Write a letter (you may or may not send) to this person, explaining why they represent integrity to you. Or make a list of the things this person has done that symbolizes integrity.
- **Recall a time when you were faced with a difficult choice** that challenged your integrity. How did you respond? What were the results? What part did God play (or not play) in this situation?
- **Find a song that encourages you in this process.** You may document the lyr-

ics and record your own reflections on them, or you could illustrate them with sketches or images you locate. Two examples for this week's study are "Integrity" by River Valley Worship (2021) and "Undivided Heart" by Davy Flowers (2022).

Your journal holds a very private and personal process; therefore, share it carefully. If social media is a healthy place for you, use these hashtags for posting your words, images, other reflections, or personal stories from this study: #fp4h and #fp4hfitforaking. You can view my journal and others' entries using these hashtags.

Help me, Lord, to follow You with integrity today. I am tempted to make choices that would compromise my faithfulness to You and I need Your help to choose Your way, not mine. Forgive me when I stumble and pick me up to continue on my journey of fitness and wellness as I seek You first. Amen.

1 "What does the Bible say about integrity?" Got Questions? (2022), https://www.gotquestions.org/Bible-integrity.html.

2 David Guzik, "Study Guide for Psalm 101," Blue Letter Bible (2002), https://www.blueletterbible.org/comm/guzik_david/study-guide/psalm/psalm-101.cfm%20.

3 "May 5, 2005: The Day Andy Roddick's Sportsmanship Cost Him a Win," Tennis Majors (2023), https://www.tennismajors.com/our-features/on-this-day/may-5-2005-the-day-andy-roddicks-sportsmanship-cost-him-victory-210307.html.

4 "Allen V. Astin–A Legacy of Integrity," National Institute for Standards and Technology (2018), https://www.nist.gov/speech-testimony/allen-v-astin-legacy-integrity.

5 Daniel Taylor, "Letters to My Children," Bog Walk Press: 2010, retrieved from Illustration Ideas, https://illustrationideas.bible/integrity/.

WEEK SIX: DAVID'S REBELLION

SCRIPTURE MEMORY VERSE
Create in me a pure heart, O God, and renew a steadfast spirit within me. Psalm 51:10

Anakin Skywalker started out as a good person in the beginning of the Star Wars saga. He was trained to become a Jedi, strongly connected to the Force, and seemed to be the fulfillment of the prophesy about the Chosen One. He had everything going for him. But he had a fatal flaw. He was afraid of loss, and it caused him to join the dark side of the Force and become Darth Vader, one of the most feared villains in literature and movies.

Up to this point in our study, *Fit for a King*, David followed God faithfully. But like all of us, he was not perfect. He defeated a giant but he also committed gigantic sins. Although he had a fatal flaw, he was still fit to be king. God did not remove him from the throne as He had done with King Saul. What was different about David? And what can we learn from him that can help us when we also rebel against God and go our own way?

In last week's *Fit for a King* study we learned about David's integrity.
*   David demonstrated integrity in his relationship to those in authority over him.
*   David did not manipulate his way into the kingship and remembered his covenant with Jonathan to care for his family.
*   When he and his troops faced a crisis, David maintained his integrity.
*   David's integrity extended to the way he handled resources.
*   David practiced integrity throughout his lifetime and modeled it for his son Solomon, the next king.

This week we will dive into the times that David rebelled against God. We can follow how David came to the point where he rejected God's plan for him at critical points in his life and how he came back to Him. This affirms there is hope for us when we don't obey God, and we can be restored to a right relationship with Him no matter what we have done. When we make unhealthy choices with food, it is not the end of our story. The King of Kings has provided a way for us to receive forgiveness for our failures and be free from harmful behaviors through His Son Jesus, our Savior.

—— DAY 1: BATHSHEBA

I open my heart to You, Father, and pray that You would speak to me through Your Word. I still have much to learn about following You with my whole being.

Just as the slaying of Goliath is David's most famous victory, his sin with Bathsheba and the aftermath of that sin is his most famous failure. How did David, the man with a heart after God and fit to be king, commit such horrific acts?

Turn to 2 Samuel 11 and read verse 1. What did David do in the spring of that year and what was unusual about what he did?

He abandoned leadership of his army and didn't take them into battle as usual. We don't know why he stayed behind. There could have been a legitimate reason for his choice to remain in Jerusalem. Whatever the reason, however, he found himself in a vulnerable position because he was not on the field of battle with his troops. Where was David in verse 2 and what did he see?

Making poor choices sometimes starts with where we are. If I'm at a party and unhealthy food choices are calling to me from the refreshment table, I can avoid going near it. If I'm at the grocery store, I can circumvent the cookie aisle because I don't want to take them home with me. If I have a choice about the restaurant where I will eat, I can choose one that has healthier options for that day's food plan. I find more success with making healthy choices when I limit my access to food that entices me to overeat or eat what's not the best for me. How do you handle keeping yourself out of tempting situations?

David found himself confronted with a choice. He could have stopped looking at the woman and gone back into the palace. But his lust got the better of his sound judgment. His second mistake was staying on the roof and continuing to look at Bathsheba. Look at 2 Samuel 11:3-4. What did David do?

_____

_____

_____

It is important to note that Bathsheba was a victim in this situation. It was customary for people of this time period to bathe on rooftops, and David would have known. She did not have a choice about sleeping with the king who sent for her. "David's lustful craving [was] coupled with an abuse of his power."[1] What was the result of David's actions (verse 5)?

_____

_____

_____

The progression of David's choices parallel James 1:14-15. Read these verses and fidentify the steps of progression that temptation takes.

First _____

Second _____

Finally _____

James's imagery of new life beginning is in stark contrast to the death created by sin. We do not have to give in to sin, however. Read Matthew 26:41. What did Jesus say is a preventative measure we can take before temptation strikes us?

_____

_____

_____

This instruction from Jesus is especially poignant because He was praying, "My Father, if it is possible, may this cup be taken from me. Yet not as I will, but as you will." (verse 7) In fact, Matthew records that He said the prayer three times.

David's third mistake is that he didn't turn to God in prayer when he was faced with temptation. Prayer is an integral part of our First Place for Health practices. We pray for ourselves and for our group members because we know prayer to the all-powerful God makes a difference. One of the most important results of prayer is the change that happens within the person who is praying. She releases her will to God and submits to His authority. The one who is on her knees in the Father's presence has more power to overcome temptation. He is faithful to provide whatever we need to say "No" to unhealthy choices and yes to Him (1 Corinthians 10:13).

How does prayer help you handle temptation?

_____

_____

_____

God, give me victory over temptation in my life, especially with my food and exercise choices. I cannot overcome temptation in my own power. I want to fully experience the freedom I have in Christ as I submit my will to Yours. Amen.

——— DAY 2: URIAH
Today is another day for me to choose to follow You fully, O Father. Use Your Word to fill me with Your power and presence.

After David learned that Bathsheba was pregnant with his child, he could have come clean and confessed his sin. But he made his next mistake by trying to hide what he had done. In 2 Samuel 11:6, David called Bathsheba's husband Uriah back from the battlefield. From 2 Samuel 23:24-39 we learn Uriah was a member of the elite group of David's army known as the Thirty, men who had risen in the ranks due to their great achievements in battle. He was a Hittite, which meant he chose to leave his nation and culture and become part of the Jewish community. Surely David knew him and had fought alongside him. Perhaps he had enlisted Uriah to join his troops during his time of running from King Saul. What did David say to Uriah in 2 Samuel 11:7-8?

_____

_____

_____

What did Uriah do in verse 9?

_____

_____

_____

Look at verses 10-13. What did David try to do next?

_____

_____

_____

When his plans to get Uriah to sleep with his wife failed, what did David instruct Joab to do to Uriah (verses 14-17)?

_____

_____

_____

Uriah demonstrated more integrity than David, who covered up his sin and abused his military power in order to have one of his best men killed. In verses 26-27, what was the aftermath of Uriah's death?

_____

_____

_____

What does verse 27 say about God's view of David's actions?

_____

_____

_____

David thought he had gotten away with adultery and murder. Did he have peace in his heart? I can't imagine that he did, a man deeply devoted to God before this event, who loved God and depended on Him through many dark days in his life. He knew God was aware of his sin and he knew God was displeased. Yet he managed to go on with his life, his new wife, and baby without acknowledging his sin to himself or God. But God was not done with David. He spoke to him through the prophet Nathan, who told David a story about a rich man who stole a beloved lamb from his neighbor to make it into a meal. How interesting that God chose a story about a lamb to gain sympathy from the former shepherd. David angrily pronounced judgment on the rich man, saying he should pay back his neighbor four times what he took. What did Nathan say to David in 2 Samuel 12:7-12?

_____

_____

_____

What was David's response in 2 Samuel 12:13?

_____

_____

_____

What would God do (verses 13-14)?

_____

_____

_____

At last David confronted his sin and showed great remorse for what he had done. He immediately responded honestly that he had sinned, not making excuses or trying to hide anything. Until he honestly confessed his sin, he could not find forgiveness and a restored relationship with God. There would be consequences for his sin, including constant family conflicts (verse 10). His baby would die (verse 13). But he would continue to be king of Israel because God knew his heart was still fit to be a king. One horrific mistake did not end David's story, just as sin in our lives doesn't end ours. When we make poor choices with food and don't confront what we've done, we are likely to continue that pattern of eating. Some of us struggle with overeating in secret. The way to change our behavior to get it out in the open. Write what you eat in your tracker, talk to a trusted friend or counselor, and pray to God, believing He will change you from the inside out.

Psalm 51 is David's journal entry, written after being confronted by Nathan and confessing his sin. What did David ask God to do in Psalm 51:10? This verse is our memory verse for this week. Write it here.

_____

_____

_____

Read verses 11-12. What other things does David ask God to do?

_____

_____

_____

What possible good does David see that could come from his experience (verse 13)?

_____

_____

_____

This part of David's story is a cautionary tale for us. First, don't allow temptation to overtake you. But when it does, immediately be honest about what you've done and ask God for forgiveness and help to do better. Finally, allow Him to use your experience to help others in similar circumstances. That's one purpose for the First Place for Health community. We all face struggles with food choices and maintenance of healthy patterns of living, and we share them with our fellow group members. We support each other and pray for each other. We overcome these struggles by learning from each other. Is there any sin or unhealthy practice you need to confess to God right now? If so, what is it?

_____

_____

_____

Accept the great forgiveness God offers through His Son Jesus, Who gave His life for you. You can tell Him anything and He will always love you. Our sin does not define us; we are defined by our God and His grace.

Have mercy on me, O God, according to Your unfailing love; according to Your great compassion blot out my transgressions. Wash away all my iniquity and cleanse me from my sin. Amen.

—— DAY 3: MULTIPLE MARRIAGES
I bring my problems and concerns to You, Holy Father, knowing Your patient passion for me will bring me peace. I open my heart, eyes, and ears to You as You speak gently to my heart.

In Deuteronomy 17:16-17 God gives important directions about Israel's future kings. What four things does He say the king should not do?

_____

_____

_____

David did not follow all of these directions. One in particular became a source of great conflict and sorrow in his life and for his people: marrying many wives. Why did God warn future kings about taking many wives (verse 17)?

_____

_____

_____

Turn to 2 Samuel 3:2-5. At this time David was king over the tribe of Judah and ruled from the town of Hebron. What do we learn about him and his family in these verses?

_____

_____

_____

After he became king over all Israel, he moved his family to Jerusalem. What does 2 Samuel 5:13-16 say about David?

_____

_____

_____

God had specifically said that the king should not take many wives. But David had more than eight wives plus multiple concubines (like a wife but with a lower status). And he had more than 20 children with them. Polygamy was not God's original plan for marriage (Genesis 1:26-28, 2:24). But the practice began soon after Adam and Eve were exiled from Eden. The first recorded instance is Lamech in Genesis 4:19. David had no problem taking women as wives or concubines, and we've already read about what he did with Bathsheba. We can infer that he had strong sexual desires and took advantage of his influence to satisfy them. His many sons from various wives became competitors for his attention and his throne. We will look at a few examples of their dysfunctional relationships later this week.

Revisit 2 Samuel 12:10-12. Although God forgave David's sin, what did He say would result from David's adultery and murder?

_____

_____

_____

David's sons fulfilled that prophesy with rebellion and violence. Unfortunately, his son and next king Solomon followed his father's example of polygamy. What does 1 Kings 11:1-3 say about him?

_____

_____

_____

What were the results of his actions (verses 4-5)?

_____

_____

_____

Verse 6 notes a connection; what is it?

_____

_____

_____

David set an example for his son that violated God's rules for Israel's kings, and Solomon and the nation of Israel paid a heavy price for their rebellion. David allowed his fleshly desires to become a fatal flaw that ruled his choices in this area of his life. First John 2:16 identifies three worldly influences that feed our fleshly desires; what are they?

_____

_____

_____

Find Romans 8:5-8; what two parts of our beings are fighting for control of our lives?

_____

_____

_____

According to these verses, how can we keep from giving in to our fleshly desires?

_____

_____

_____

Sexual desire is healthy and a gift from God. But David chose to feed his fleshly desires rather than follow God's plan of sex within marriage with one wife. The desire to eat is healthy. Our bodies need food for energy, function, and repair. We need balanced proportions of protein, fat, and carbohydrate nutrients in reasonable portions every day. When we focus on feeding our fleshly desires, we can easily go beyond those healthy parameters and harm our bodies. We can choose to allow our flesh to rule or we can choose to walk in the spirit and follow God's perfect plan for us. Daily communion with Him and submission to His will through the power of the Holy Spirit give us victory over our flesh. We do not have to follow in David's footsteps. Read 1 Corinthians 15:56-57 and write verse 57 here.

_____

_____

_____

Thank You, Lord, for Your Holy Spirit's indwelling in me. My desire to follow my own flesh is a constant battle, but I claim victory over sin because Jesus has already won the war. Help me to walk in triumphant freedom today. Amen.

—— DAY 4: THE CENSUS

Holy Lord, I bow before You in Your sacred presence, pleading for Your wisdom and strength during another day on earth. Without You, I am lost.

Another instance of David rebelling against God is found in 2 Samuel 24. Read verses 1-2. What did David do?

_____

_____

_____

Depending on the translation you read, verse 1 may seem to indicate that God caused David to sin. However, in the original language there is no subject in the sentence to identify who incited David to take the census. 1 Chronicles 21:1 says, "Satan rose up against Israel and incited David to take a census of Israel." Yet the subject of this sentence also is ambiguous in the original text. It could have been the enemy or a person offering David poor advice. It could have been David's own idea.[2] Whatever the case, we can be sure God was in charge, possibly testing David's faith in Him. What does James 1:13 say about temptation?

Why was taking this census an act of rebellion toward God? Cultural norms at that time said that you could only take a count of what belonged to you. The Israelite people didn't belong to David; they belonged to God. Only God could order a census of His people (Exodus 30:12, Numbers 1:1-2). David knew it was the wrong thing to do, as did his advisors. What did Joab say in 1 Chronicles 21:3?

God gave David a chance to change his mind before he committed a sin. However, David didn't answer Joab's question and insisted he and his men take the census. Why do you think David wanted to take a census?

What happened after the census had been taken (verse 10)?

How did God respond to David's prayer (verses 11-13)?

What option did David choose and why (verse 14)?

Once the plague started, what did David pray (verse 17)?

_____

_____

_____

What did the angel of the Lord order Gad to tell David what to do (verse 18)?

_____

_____

_____

We read last week about David's purchase of Araunah's threshing floor to build the altar. And God stopped the plague once David obeyed Him (verse 25). But the damage had been done. According to verse 15 over 70,000 people died before God paused the plague. He showed mercy even in His judgment and cancelled the plague before an entire day had passed. David was wise to trust God and not other people for his punishment. We may be left wondering why God would allow innocent people to die for David's sin. But He doesn't give us a reason, much like the story of Job's suffering. These stories emphasize the choice we continually face: trust God or trust someone or something else. The result is always the same: *trusting God is best*. When we don't trust God and act in our own prideful ways, we open ourselves up for consequences that can be mild or massive. Other people can be hurt by our rebellion and we can be hurt by other people's rebellion. That is not the way God wanted His world to operate from the beginning, but once sin entered the world through human beings' prideful choices, His perfect creation became corrupted. What do the following scripture references teach us about pride?

Scripture	What It Says about Pride
Proverbs 11:2	
Proverbs 18:12	
Galatians 6:3	
James 4:6	

Read Jeremiah 9:23-24. What does God tell us not to boast about in verse 23?

_____

_____

_____

What does verse 24 say we should boast about?

_____

_____

_____

When you are faced with a choice between satisfying your pride or trusting God, stop and think about the greatness of God and how much He has done for you. If you are tempted to make an unhealthy food choice, turn to Him and sing His praises! Our God is amazing in power and love, and we can trust Him wholeheartedly to always do what is best for us, even when we don't understand. He is always with us and will guide us into His right paths if we will count on Him.

Father, help me to choose to praise You when I am tempted by my pride. You are the great and mighty King of all creation Who brings salvation and healing to all who choose to call on You. Amen.

—— DAY 5: LAZY LEADERSHIP AND PASSIVE PARENTING
I am looking to You alone for the strength to face another day, precious Lord. You know the challenges I will face and the battles I will fight. Use this quiet time to fill me with Your wisdom and truth.

Another area of his life where David did not follow God fully was in his leadership, both with his army and with his sons. First let's look at Joab, the head of his army. Read 1 Chronicles 2:13-16 and identify his relationship to David.

_____

_____

_____

In 1 Chronicles 11:4-9 we learn how Joab became David's general over his army. What battle did Joab win for David?

_____

_____

_____

We read about Joab last week when we looked at David's treatment of King Saul's general Abner. Joab killed Abner because Abner had killed Joab's brother, although Abner had done it in self-defense (2 Samuel 3:27). What was David's response to Joab's murder of Abner (2 Samuel 3:28-29, 39)?

_____

_____

_____

David condemned the act and cursed Joab, but he didn't punish Joab in any way. In fact, Abner's murder took place before Joab conquered the Jebusites, took what became the city that became Jerusalem, and was promoted to leader of David's army.

David also showed passivity in parenting his sons. His oldest son Amnon raped his half-sister Tamar (2 Samuel 13:1-22). How did David respond to this violent act (verse 21)?

_____

_____

_____

Two years later Tamar's brother Absalom schemed to take revenge on Amnon. David gave his permission for Absalom to have a dinner with Amnon as a guest, and it was there that Amnon was killed. When David learned of Amnon's murder (first reported as the murder of all his sons), what did David do (2 Samuel 13:31)?

_____

_____

_____

Absalom fled the country but later returned at David's invitation. Yet David refused to see his son for two years and never enacted any punishment for him killing his half-brother. Absalom eventually tried to overthrow his father's rule. When the battle for control took place, David told Joab to "Be gentle with the young man Absalom for my sake" (2 Samuel 18:5). Read 2 Samuel 18:14-15 to find out what Joab did.

_____

_____

_____

General Joab also killed his cousin Amasa (another nephew of David) whom Absalom had put in charge of his own army (2 Samuel 20:9-10). When David was on his death-bed he instructed his son Solomon concerning Joab. Find 1 Kings 2:5-6 and record what he told Solomon to do with Joab and why.

_____

_____

_____

What pattern do you notice about David's reactions to each of these circumstances?

_____

_____

_____

David tended to be passive in his relationships with others rather than being forceful. He didn't discipline his general or his sons when they needed it. He let Joab continue to lead the army even after he murdered Abner, Absalom, and Amasa, all relatives. He didn't discipline Amnon for raping Tamar, and he foolishly allowed Absalom to invite Amnon to an event where he could have him killed. David's grief over his son Absalom's death almost cost him his army's loyalty (2 Samuel 19:1-8). He waited so long to make his son Solomon king that a vacuum of power existed, enabling his son Adonijah to attempt a coup. First Kings 1:6 says, "His father had never rebuked [Adonijah} by asking, 'Why do you behave as you do?'" David's desire to avoid conflict in his personal and professional relationships allowed others to literally get away with murder.

What is the lesson for us? We should confront conflict sooner than later. David saw Joab's violent tendency before he made him leader of his army, but he gave him the leadership anyway and continued to verbally condemn his murderous actions without holding him accountable. His hands-off approach in correcting his sons clearly gave them confidence to do anything they wanted. David's decisions to ignore these un-pleasant situations reveals laziness in leadership. He didn't want to do corrective tasks that were unpleasant to him when dealing with relational conflicts.

When we allow uncomfortable situations to go unresolved, they don't go away. They just get worse. If you are struggling with issues that influence you to make unhealthy choices, your behavior will not significantly or permanently change until you confront the issues. Don't ignore the conflict. Face the truth and take the needed action. Do the hard work now or you will find there is harder work to do in the long run. "The destruction brought about by avoiding the conflict is many times worse than the unpleasantness that might have resulted from dealing with the issues when they first arose."[3] Conflicts and hurt emotions will not heal on their own. Processing painful emotions that we'd rather avoid is worth the effort.

Are there any areas in your life where you are avoiding conflict? If so, what are they?

Don't abandon your responsibility to God, others, and yourself by ignoring difficult situations and putting them off until later. Ask God for wisdom and strength to face uncomfortable conflicts and stand strong with His help.

I confess I'd rather not face conflicts but avoid them. I need to be proactive and not passive in my relationships with others. Give me courage to handle these situations and make healthy choices for myself and others. Amen.

—— DAY 6: REFLECTION AND APPLICATION

In this quiet moment, Holy Lord, I turn my face away from worldly worries and distracted thinking so I may fully abide in Your presence. I'm listening for Your words of healing and hope.

Practice reciting this week's memory verse by writing it here.

When I was in eighth grade my church hired its first youth director, who also served as our new music minister. He was a young man with a wife and two small daughters. He developed a thriving youth and music ministry in our church. I grew in so many ways during the years he led our church. But his tenure at our church had a tragic end. He became involved with a young woman in our youth group. He was dismissed from our church and his marriage dissolved. It was a devastating time for our church, his family, and me personally, as I had looked up to him and depended on him as a strong, faithful spiritual leader. I saw first-hand the gut-retching consequences of sexual sin on the leader who committed it as well as the far-reaching ripple effects that his actions caused.

David's adultery and murderous scheme affected his family and the nation of Israel in many horrific ways. He tried to hide his sin but was unsuccessful. He confessed and repented, but the consequences still hurt him and others for many years. His writing in Psalm 51 indicated his deep regret and sorrow over his sin, not because of the consequences, but because he knew he had sacrificed his intimacy with God. His sexual desire proved to be his fatal flaw.

Ancient Greek writers began the tradition of using heroes with fatal flaws in their plays and poems. The word they used for this type of character trope was *hamartia*. It means to miss the mark, like aiming an arrow at a target and missing the bullseye. This is the same word used in the New Testament to describe sin: *hamartia*. It is "forfeiture because (of) missing the mark" and "the brand of sin that emphasizes its self-originated (self-empowered) nature—-i.e., it is not originated or empowered by God."[4] We are all born with the fatal flaw of missing the mark, and we must wrestle with it constantly. But God has given us power over sin through Jesus's death and resurrection. We do not have to succumb to the fatal flaw of sin. We can live in freedom and victory over it.

We started the week with these two questions: what was different about David's responses to his own rebellion and what can we learn from him that can help us when we rebel? One difference is David was quick to confess and repent from sin in most cases. Next week we will dive deeper into this humble attitude. God was able to continue using him as the leader of Israel, even though he was not perfect. What other differences did you notice about David this week?

_____

_____

_____

What is the most important lesson that you have learned or revisited from this week's study of David's rebellion? How does that lesson relate to your life, now or in the past?

_____

_____

_____

Thank You for David, God, and for teaching me about rebellion through his life. I admit I am faced with choices every day that tempt me to rebel and do my will instead of Yours. I commit anew to putting You first in all things and submitting to Your Lordship. Thank You for forgiveness and salvation. Amen.

—— DAY 7: REFLECTION AND APPLICATION

I seek You today, Father, for all that I need. My life is open before You as we meet now, and I ask You to flood me with Your power and presence.

Reading about David's rebellion this week may have been difficult. Sin and its aftermath is not an uplifting topic. But knowing that sin is preventable and forgivable is the hope we have as followers of Christ. God is able to give us victory over our sin and is ready to forgive us when we miss the mark. As you reflect on these ideas today, ask God to show you where you need repentance and accept His wonderful gift of forgiveness. Here are some prompts to help you with that process.

- **Think about a time when you made an unhealthy food choice.** What were the things that happened before you put the food in your mouth? Write down each step that brought you to that point. Identify anything that you could have done differently. How can this knowledge help you to make better choices in the future?
- **Meditate on Psalm 51:1-15.** Select words and phrases that are meaningful to you and record them in your journal. Use this journal entry with your prayers to remind you to confess your sins to God and receive His forgiveness. You may include other scriptures such as 1 John 1:9 in your journaling.
- **How do you deal with conflict** in your personal and professional relationships? Do you confront difficult situations or do you avoid them? Identify a conflict that needs your attention and develop a plan for facing that conflict. Ask God to show you what you need to do to bring the conflict to a resolution as much as it depends on you. Enlist the help of a trusted friend or counselor if needed.
- **Find a song that encourages you** in this process. You may document the lyrics and record your own reflections on them, or you could illustrate them with sketches or images you locate. Two examples for this week's study are "Forgive Me, Lord" by Surgenor Music (2014) and "Create in Me a Clean Heart" by Keith Green (1990).

Your journal holds a very private and personal process; therefore, share it carefully. If social media is a healthy place for you, use these hashtags for posting your words, images, other reflections, or personal stories from this study: #fp4h and #fp4hfit-foraking. You can view my journal and others' entries using these hashtags.

Oh God, my heart is full of love and gratitude for the amazing salvation You provide for me through my Lord Jesus Christ. I am redeemed by the blood of the Lamb and I am walking in victory through Your Holy Spirit's power. I rejoice in the freedom You give me every day. Amen.

1 Leslie Vernick, "A New Way of Seeing David's Sin with Bathsheba," Leslie Vernick & Co. (2010), https://leslievernick.com/blog/a-new-way-of-seeing-davids-sin-with-bathsheba/#:~:text=David%20 took%20Bathsheba%20to%20his,2%20Samuel%2011%20and%2012).

2 "Why Was God So Angry at David for Taking the Census?" Got Questions, https://www.gotques-tions.org/David-census.html.

3 "David's Dysfunctional Handling of Family Conflict Leads to Civil War (2 Samuel 13-19)," Theology of Work Project, https://www.theologyofwork.org/old-testament/samuel-kings-chronicles-and-work/ the-golden-age-of-the-monarchy-2-samuel-1-24-1-kings-1-11-1-chronicles-21-2/davids-successes-and-failures-as-king-2-samuel-1-24/davids-dysfunctional-handling-of-family-conflict-leads-to-civ-il-war-2-samue.

4 Strong's Concordance, Bible Hub (2021), https://biblehub.com/greek/266.htm.

WEEK SEVEN: DAVID'S HUMILITY

SCRIPTURE MEMORY VERSE
For he knows how we are formed, he remembers that we are dust. Psalm 103:14

Nelson Mandela became president of South Africa in 1944, the first black leader elected to this position. He took office after the end of apartheid, a policy that discriminated against nonwhite minorities, a policy he and his organization helped to destroy. On his first day as president, he didn't see any of the staff in the office. He called a meeting of all staff members for the next day. When he entered the room where they were waiting for him, he looked around at their faces. It was easy to sense the antagonism of some of the staffers who were meeting their new black president and boss for the first time. He approached the person nearest him. He asked if he could shake her hand and began asking questions, including her name, marital status, and whether or not she had any children. He continued this process until he had greeted every person individually, which took him over an hour to accomplish. After a few months, every staff member was won over and embraced him and his leadership.[1] Mandela did not use his powerful position to dominate over his subordinates. Instead he was humble in his relations with his staff and everyone he met. His humility contributed to one of the greatest revolutions in history.

Last week's study of *Fit for a King* we identified times when David rebelled against God.
- David committed adultery by making a series of bad choices.
- David had Uriah killed in order to cover up his sin, compounding his rebellion.
- God commanded that Israel's kings should not take many wives, but David had at least 20 wives and concubines.
- When David ordered a census of the people, he violated God's law and revealed his pride, resulting in thousands of deaths.
- David's passive attitude in personal and professional relationships caused serious problems for him and his people.

A case can be made that all of David's rebellious acts were rooted in pride, believing his way was better than God's. Humility is the antithesis of pride. Throughout most of his life, David practiced humility, bowing before God's sovereignty and trusting Him alone. And even when he rebelled, he responded in humility to God's discipline. How can we develop and maintain an attitude of humility and follow God faithfully, especially in our food and exercise choices? We'll look at David, God's choice to be Israel's king, to discover his humble heart and reflect on who sits on the throne of our hearts: ourselves or God.

—— DAY 1: HUMILITY AND THANKFULNESS
What a gift to have a quiet time alone with You, my Father. Help me to put aside all things that distract me from listening to You and finding all I need in Your presence.

Write this week's memory verse here.

_____

_____

_____

The word *humility* comes from a word for earth or dirt. There isn't anything much lowlier in the world than dirt! This etymology provides a better understanding of the concept of humility and the imagery of dirt in our memory verse. One writer says,

> A speck of dust does not think itself more superior or inferior than another, nor does it concern itself for what other specks of dust might or might not think. Enthralled by the miracle of existence, the truly humble person lives not for herself or her image, but for life itself, in a condition of pure peace and pleasure.[2]

Unfortunately our human tendency is pride, which is the opposite of humility. C.S. Lewis describes pride this way:

> According to Christian teachers, the essential vice, the utmost evil, is Pride. Unchastity, anger, greed, drunkenness, and all that, are mere flea bites in comparison: it was through Pride that the devil became the devil: Pride leads to every other vice: it is the *complete anti-God state of mind*...it is Pride which has been the chief cause of misery in every nation and every family since the world began (emphasis added).[3]

This attitude contrasts sharply with humility. God needed a ruler who would fully submit to Him so He could lead His people through him. King Saul lacked this humility and it caused his downfall. David was different; he was humble before his God.

Developing a consistently humble mindset takes time and intentional work to coun-
teract pride. One way to stimulate humility is through thankfulness. When we thank
God for His character and His blessings, we position ourselves under His authority.
We recognize all good things come from Him and not ourselves. David wrote many
psalms of thankfulness. Turn to Psalm 100. What did David invite us to do in verses
1-2?

_____

_____

_____

How does verse 3 convey the idea of humility?

_____

_____

_____

What two things did David encourage us to do as we enter God's presence (verse 4)?

_____

_____

_____

What characteristics of God did David call to our attention in verse 5?

_____

_____

_____

Read 1 Chronicles 16:34-36, part of David's prayer during the Ark of the Covenant's
glorious return to Jerusalem. Why should we give thanks to the Lord, according to
verse 34?

_____

_____

_____

In verse 35 what did David ask God to do to allow His people to thank and praise
Him?

_____

_____

_____

What characteristics of God did David call to our attention in verse 36?

_____

_____

_____

Both of these passages point out an important characteristic of God: He is eternal. He never ends. Is there anything or anyone else that can claim this quality? God's eternal nature give us assurance that we need in a world where everything seems ephemeral and disposable. As I thank God for all the good things in my life, I recognize that His eternal nature will continue to provide for me now and in the future. When I have a humble attitude, it is easy to be thankful because I know my blessings are not from my own efforts but a result of God's grace. I can thank God for the healthy food He provides for me to eat rather than complain about avoiding food that is less healthy for me.

For what would you like to thank God right now? Write a prayer of thanksgiving to Him here.

_____

_____

_____

Thank You, Father, for Your amazing generosity toward me. I am grateful for everything You give me. I praise Your eternal nature that gives me strength to face each day, knowing You will never leave me or forsake me. Amen.

—— DAY 2: HUMILITY AND REPENTANCE

In the presence of the Lord there is peace. In You alone I find hope and security. No foe can stand against me as long as You are my strength and shield.

How do you respond when someone criticizes you? Most of us get defensive. We might respond with excuses or try to point out something negative about the person criticizing us. It is not easy to hear that we might be less than perfect, and our human tendency toward prideful attitudes wants to deny any flaw in our characters or actions.

When was the last time someone pointed out a mistake you made or criticized you for some reason? What did they say and how did you respond?

We have seen several situations in David's life when he was confronted by his sinfulness and mistakes. He accepted responsibility for his actions without trying to shift blame or make excuses. When he was confronted about his sin with Bathsheba and Uriah, he said, "*I have sinned* against the Lord" (2 Samuel 12:13, emphasis added). When he realized he had sinned by taking the census he said, "*I have sinned* greatly in what I have done. Now, LORD, I beg you, take away the guilt of your servant. I have done a very foolish thing" (2 Samuel 24:10, emphasis added). His humility is evident in his immediate recognition and confession of his sin to God.

Last week we read part of Psalm 51, which David wrote after he confessed his sin with Bathsheba and Uriah. He humbly confessed to God in verses 3-4, "I know my transgressions, and my sin is always before me. Against you, you only, have I sinned and done what is evil in your sight." Let's look at another psalm David wrote about repentance. Find Psalm 32. What characteristics did David list in verses 1-2 for the person who is blessed? There are at least four.

What happened to David when he kept silent about his sin (verse 3-4)?

In verse 5 what did David do and how did God respond?

Read the rest of the psalm, verses 6-11. What did David say we should do in verse 6 and how does that help us (verses 6-7)?

_____

_____

_____

In verses 8-9 God said, "I will instruct you and teach you in the way you should go; I will counsel you with my loving eye on you." What did God warn us against in verse 10?

_____

_____

_____

How did David end the psalm in verse 11? How does that contrast with verse 4?

_____

_____

_____

One of David's descendants, King Uzziah, chose pride over humility. Look up 2 Chronicles 26. In verses 4-5 we read that Uzziah was a good king who followed God faithfully. However, what happened in verse 16?

_____

_____

_____

Only priests were allowed to burn incense in the temple. The priests confronted King Uzziah but he ignored them. As a result of his pride, what happened to him in verses 19-20?

_____

_____

_____

The affliction lasted the rest of his life, forced him to live in a separate house, and excluded him from the temple. He started strong in his faithfulness to God, but pride became his downfall. This story warns us to be alert to sin and confess it humbly as soon as we become aware of it. Pride is a barrier to repentance and forgiveness, but humility is a door.

Is there any pride in your life that needs to be brought before the Lord? If so, take time now to pray to God, humbly and honestly admitting it and receiving His abundant forgiveness in Christ Jesus. Write in your journal if you wish.

My loving Lord, I am guilty of sin. Every day I must face the truth that I cannot live a perfect life. Help me to humbly bring my flaws and failures to You for repentance and forgiveness. I want to walk in Your ways consistently as I continue to seek You first. Amen.

—— DAY 3: HUMILITY AND ACCEPTANCE

I bow before the Lord my God, my Maker and Redeemer. You are the reason I live and the song in my heart. I desire to serve You with my whole being.

After David had been confronted about his sin with Bathsheba and Uriah, the prophet Nathan told him that the child born from his adulterous act would die. David's response to that news reveals another aspect of his humility. Read 2 Samuel 12:15-17. What did David do when the child became ill?

_____

_____

_____

What happened on the seventh day (verses 18-19)?

_____

_____

_____

What does verse 20 say about David's response to the news about his child?

_____

_____

_____

In verse 21 David's attendants questioned him about his behavior. How did David answer them in verse 22?

_____

_____

_____

Job had a similar response to the tragedies that struck him, tragedies that were not a result of his own sin. What did he say in Job 1:20?

_____

_____

_____

Both David and Job recognized the sovereignty of God. They understood that His decisions are final and inscrutable. They trusted Him even in the midst of pain and loss, and although they were grieving, they humbly accepted their situations. They turned toward God, not away from Him. When the apostle Paul suffered from "a thorn in the flesh," he prayed for God to remove it. But God said He would not. What did God tell Paul in 2 Corinthians 12:9?

_____

_____

_____

What is Paul's humble response to God's decision (verse 9-10)?

_____

_____

_____

Acceptance of difficulties does not mean we don't feel grief and pain because of our circumstances. There is no sin in emotional sorrow. But spiritually and mentally we can accept what happens because we know God is in control and will never leave us or forsake us. Peter wrote about how we can respond to suffering because of our relationship to Christ. What did he say in 1 Peter 4:12-13?

_____

_____

_____

Notice we suffer for Christ's glory, once again encouraging us to remain humble. In verses 16 and 19, what did Peter say we should do that represents humility?

_____

_____

_____

Everyone suffers difficulties, whether they are Christians or not, whether they caused the suffering or not. It is a human condition. How we respond to our suffering reveals our character and who sits on the throne of our lives. We can constantly complain and have a continuous pity party or we can humbly bow before God and accept what we have experienced. We can whine that losing weight is hard and that we don't want to make healthy choices to accomplish our goals. Or we can accept the challenge to submit our desires and habits to God and become our healthiest selves under the leadership and power of His Holy Spirit. Is there some difficulty that you need to bring before God and ask for His help to accept it?

_____

_____

_____

Recently I observed my brother-in-law showing his four-year-old granddaughter how to water the plants in his big backyard. He went with her to a bucket full of water he had mixed with plant food and demonstrated how to dip the liquid into a container. Then he walked with her and showed her where to pour it on the first group of plants. He walked back with her to get more water and went with her to the next group of plants. He continued to walk alongside her again and again until all the plants were watered. I was reminded about the way God walks alongside us, showing us how to live, taking every step with us. He does not tell us what to do in His Word then sit back to see how we will handle ourselves in difficulties. He is right beside us, walking through the valleys with us, strengthening and encouraging us. This knowledge helps us accept our trials as David, Job, and Paul accepted their trials. We can live free from despair and depression over trying times because we know our loving God is with us.

Your presence in my pain gives me strength and hope, Lord. Your passion for me encourages me to turn to You during difficult times. Help me accept what You have allowed me to experience, knowing that when I am humble and meek, You can accomplish mighty acts in and through me. Amen.

—— DAY 4: HUMILITY AND SERVANTHOOD
I want to serve You with my whole heart, Lord, but my selfish desires tend to creep into my focus. Use this time alone with You to starve my flesh and feed my spirit.

Servant leadership has been a trend in the corporate world for several decades. The concept includes putting others first and working side-by-side with employees to create a culture of team work and productivity. One example is Herb Kelleher, the founder of Southwest Airlines, who in the 1960s began a company that became known for its employee-friendly culture and customer-focused business. Herb didn't sit back in his office barking orders to his subordinates. He was shoulder-to-shoulder with his employees and created an atmosphere of mutual respect and fun. David also exemplified this model of servant leadership. Before he became king, he saw himself as a minor player in King Saul's reign. Read 1 Samuel 26:20, which took place during one of Saul's pursuits of David in the wilderness. What did David say about himself?

_____

_____

_____

Find Psalm 131:1. What does King David say about himself?

_____

_____

_____

When God revealed His plan to David to keep his descendants on the throne of His kingdom, how did David respond? Find the answer in 2 Samuel 18:19.

_____

_____

_____

One of David's descendants, Jesus, lived the ultimate life of servant leadership. Read John 13:2-5 and describe His act of humility.

_____

_____

_____

What did Jesus want his disciples, including us, to learn from His example (verses 12-17)?

_____

_____

_____

Look up Philippians 2:5-8 and write in your own words how Jesus modeled humility.

_____

_____

_____

He died for me so I could live. And as a leader, whether in my personal relationships or my professional life, I too must have a sacrificial stance. I look out for the needs of my family members and co-workers rather than exalt myself above them. What does that look like for you?

_____

_____

_____

Is there a humble, servant leader in your life? If so, describe that person.

_____

_____

_____

For those of us who are First Place for Health leaders, our servant leadership can include listening to our members and responding with empathy rather than judgment, encouragement, providing advice, and preparing and conducting meetings that focus on them rather than ourselves. Helping others grow and achieve their personal goals is one of the best parts of being a leader. As the leader serves others, she too will grow and be successful. How will you practice being a servant leader this week?

_____

_____

_____

Father, I am so grateful that You became a servant leader to provide my salvation. You modeled that lifestyle perfectly, and Your Spirit lives in me so that I can serve others as You did. Show me where I can minister to others this week for Your glory and their benefit. Amen.

—— DAY 5: HUMILITY AND OBEDIENCE

God, I struggle sometimes with being completely obedient to You. I know You only have my best in mind but at times I think I know better. Help me develop total surrender to You, My loving Lord and compassionate Savior.

David had an enormous passion to build a temple for God, but God told him, "No." David could have demanded his own way: "Yeah, I hear you, God, but I want to build the temple myself." Instead, he thanked God for choosing his family as the rulers of Israel and expressed his submission to God's authority (2 Samuel 18:18-29). He understood that humility goes hand in hand with obedience to the One who he faithfully served.

Jesus and His first century followers spoke much about humility. How do Jesus's words in Matthew 16:24-25 combine the ideas of humility and obedience?

_____

_____

_____

You may have heard someone say, "Oh, this is the cross I must bear," referring to some trial or burden. But in this passage Jesus spoke to first-century Jews. The context for taking up one's cross was not the same as ours. For them it was the torturous method of Roman execution. Crosses were part of the physical landscape. It meant shameful, excruciating death under an oppressive foreign government's rule. Dying to self for the sake of Christ is the ultimate form of humility and obedience.

Locate James 4:4-7. In verse 4 who is an enemy of God?

_____

_____

_____

What does God jealously long for (verse 5)?

_____

_____

_____

James quotes a verse from Proverbs 3:34 in James 4:6. What is the contrast between the proud and the humble?

_____

_____

_____

In verse 7 what are we commanded to do that involves humility and obedience?

_____

_____

_____

Peter also quotes Proverbs 3:34 in 1 Peter 5:5. How does he instruct us in humility?

_____

_____

_____

In our First Place for Health ministry we submit to God through healthy eating and movement, as well as spiritual habits such as Bible study, scripture reading, Bible verse memorization, and prayer. What promise are we given about obeying God through humility in 1 Peter 5:6?

_____

_____

_____

What does Peter say in verse 7 that reminds us of God's love for us?

_____

_____

_____

Finally, Paul tells us about the practical side of humility and obedience. Read Philippians 4:12. Through his humble obedience to God, what has he learned to do?

_____

_____

_____

What is the result of this process of submitting to God (verse 13)?

_____

_____

_____

Humility leads to obedience which results in contentment and strength. That's a winning combination! Is there an area where you struggle with obedience, either in your eating, exercise, or something else? What is it and how can submitting to God help you be more consistently obedient to Him?

_____

_____

_____

My sweet Lord, I desire to obey You completely and joyfully. I cannot do it in my own strength but only in the strength You give me through submission and humility before You. I bow before You, my Creator and Lover of my soul, and commit again to take up my cross and follow You. Amen.

—— DAY 6: REFLECTION AND APPLICATION

I humbly come into Your mighty presence, Lord, asking for help and wisdom with all the areas of my life, for all my pains and struggles, confident in Your amazing grace and love.

Practice this week's memory verse.

_____

_____

_____

Finding a story about a person who exemplifies humility is hard, because humble people are by definition not in the spotlight. In fact, most people with a humble heart are uncomfortable with praise or public honor. Like David, they are self-effacing and quick to share acclaim with others, giving glory to God rather than themselves. What does Colossians 3:17 say about our motivation in life?

_____

_____

_____

Being humble does not mean we demean ourselves. It is not about how bad I am but how good God is. One writer says, "Humility is an attitude of spiritual modesty that comes from understanding our place in the larger order of things. It entails not taking our desires, successes, or failings too seriously."[14] A humble heart centers its focus on God and others, trusting Him to meet all of one's needs. How does Psalm 50:15 reflect this truth?

A humble heart is a healthy heart. In fact, it is said

> [humility] is good for us individually and for our relationships. For example, humble people handle stress more effectively and report higher levels of physical and mental well-being. They also show greater generosity, helpfulness, and gratitude— all things that can only serve to draw us closer to others.[5]

The benefits of humility are supported by science as well as the Bible. Proverbs 15:33 (ESV) says, "The fear of the Lord is instruction in wisdom, and humility comes before honor." What does this verse tell us about the benefits of humility?

What does Psalm 147:6 say God does for the humble?

Proverbs 3:34 says the LORD "shows _____ to the humble."

True humility comes from a heart that is focused on God. We can't try to be humble; it doesn't start with a behavior but with an attitude. David, the man fit for a king, was highly exalted by the people but lowly in his heart, a heart like God's. Take time to reflect on your own heart condition in regards to humility. Ask God to show you positions of pride that need to be turned over to Him and replaced with a spirit of submission. Thank Him for the benefits He provides to a humble heart. Write a prayer to Him here.

John Bunyan wrote,
>He that is down needs fear no fall,
>He that is low, no pride;
>He that is humble ever shall
>Have God to be his guide.[6]

You know my heart, Father, and all the ways my pride fights against my desire to obey You completely. Thank You for never giving up on me, for always working in me to weed out the seeds of sin, and for Your Spirit Who gives me wisdom and motivation to follow You faithfully. Amen.

—— DAY 7: REFLECTION AND APPLICATION

Today is another day to walk in Your ways with praise, O Lord. How I love You! I'm grateful to be Your child, an heir with Christ, and part of Your forever family.

As we have studied David's humble heart this week, what has God been saying to you? How has He worked through His word in your own heart to develop humility? Use today's time to reflect on these questions. Below are possible journaling prompts to guide your thoughts on humility.

- **Keep a gratitude journal for a week.** Each day write down something for which you can thank God. At the end of the week, write a prayer of thanksgiving and praise to God. How did this practice encourage your humility? Consider continuing this practice if you find it beneficial.
- **Read Luke 18:9–14,** Jesus's parable about the prayers of a Pharisee and a publican. Compare the two prayers and identify how this parable teaches us about humility. Which of the two people best reflects your prayers to God? Why?
- **By some accounts, there are more than seventy Bible verses about humility** and over fifty about pride. What do you think this means in regards to God's wise instruction about humility? What are some verses about humility that are most meaningful to you? There are many from this week's lesson you can choose or find other ones for your reflection. You can include images with the verses.
- **John R.W. Stott wrote, "Pride is your greatest enemy,** humility is your greatest friend."[7] Write a friendship letter to Humility and/or write a breakup letter to Pride.
- **Find a song that encourages you** in this process. You may document the lyrics and record your own reflections on them, or you could illustrate them with sketches or images you locate. Two examples for this week's study are "How Great is Our God" by Chris Tomlin (2004) and "Humble Heart" by Matt Mc-Chlery (2020).

Your journal holds a very private and personal process; therefore, share it carefully. If social media is a healthy place for you, use these hashtags for posting your words, images, other reflections, or personal stories from this study: #fp4h and #fp4hfitforaking. You can view my journal and others' entries using these hashtags.

Make my heart a humble place for Your Spirit to live and move. All I am is Yours, Father, and I rejoice in Your majesty and power. You are the one great God, the Creator and Sustainer of all life and love. Amen.

1 Pippa Green, "Mandela's Humility," Nieman Reports (2013), https://niemanreports.org/articles/mandelas-humility/.

2 Neel Burton, "What's the Difference between Modesty and Humility?" Psychology Today (2018), https://www.psychologytoday.com/us/blog/hide-and-seek/201806/whats-the-difference-between-modesty-and-humility.

3 C.S. Lewis, Mere Christianity (New York: Simon & Schuster, 1996), 109, 111.

4 Anna Katharina Schaffner, "What is Humility & Why Is It Important?" Positive Psychology (2020), https://positivepsychology.com/humility/.

5 Vicki Zakrzewski, "How Humility Will Make You the Greatest Person Ever," Greater Good Magazine (2016),
https://greatergood.berkeley.edu/article/item/humility_will_make_you_greatest_person_ever.

6 John Bunyan, The Pilgrim's Progress and Other Selected Works by John Bunyan (Green Forest AR: Master Books, 2005), 286.

7 John R. W. Stott, "Pride, Humility, and God" (Downers Grove IL: InterVarsity Press, 1992), 119, as qtd. by Thomas A. Tarrants, "Pride and Humility," C.S. Lewis Institute (2011), https://cslewisinstitute.org/resources/pride-and-humility/.

WEEK EIGHT: DAVID'S LEGACY

SCRIPTURE MEMORY VERSE
I am the Root and the Offspring of David, and the bright Morning Star.
Revelation 22:16

Barbara Jordan was an amazing woman. Her distinctive voice commanded attention, and she devoted much of her life to government service and civil rights advocacy. She served on the House Judiciary Committee that oversaw President Nixon's impeachment trial and spoke at the 1976 Democratic National Convention, significant accomplishments for one of the first two black women elected to the U.S. House of Representatives. After leaving the House, she served on the faculty of the University of Texas. When she died in 1996, she was the first black woman buried in the Texas State Cemetery in Austin. She could have requested any number of accolades to appear on her tombstone. But she asked for only one word to be inscribed: "Teacher." Of all her achievements, that role was most important to her. Her students who continue her dedication to service and justice are her legacy.

What legacy do you want to leave? How will you be remembered after you are gone? What defines your life? As Christians, we want to be known for authentically following Jesus and being His hands and feet to others. We know that the eternal awards we receive will be our heavenly crowns that we will worshipfully place at the feet of Jesus (1 Peter 5:4, Revelation 4:10-11). And we yearn to hear God's "well done, good and faithful servant" as we enter into His heavenly kingdom, forever to be with Him (Matthew 25:23).

For last week's study on *Fit for a King*, we examined David's humility.
- Thankfulness is one way to diminish pride and develop humility.
- Repentance from sin and pride requires humility.
- Humility includes understanding God works in life's circumstances to accomplish His will as He walks alongside us through every step.
- A servant mindset and lifestyle come from an attitude of humility.
- Humility goes hand in hand with obeying God.

David left an amazing legacy after living a life devoted to God. His stories and words fill the Old Testament more than any person, and he is mentioned in the New Testament as well. His presence is second only to Jesus in the scriptures. What words would have been put on his tombstone that represented his legacy? This week as we wrap up this study, *Fit for a King*, we will investigate David's legacy and consider connections to our lives. It's never too early to contemplate how your life affects others, especially in the cause for Christ and His mission to save the world. And every daily step we take to reach our goals to seek God first and love Him with all our beings, including our food and movement choices, contribute to that legacy.

—— DAY 1: ROYALTY
Because of Jesus, I am a child of the King. You are my King, O Lord, and I open my heart to You as I enter into a quiet time of studying Your precious Word.

King David left a legacy of royalty for his descendants. Every king of Judah after David was his progeny. Some of them followed God and some didn't, but all of them knew about David's life and his commitment to Yahweh. Let's identify some of the kings who followed David and learn about their legacies. Look up the scriptures in the chart. Record the name of each king and at least one thing he accomplished.

Scripture	King's Name	Accomplishment
1 Chronicles 14:2-6		
2 Kings 17:1-6		
2 Chronicles 29:1-2, 18-19, 31:1		
2 Chronicles 34:1-3, 8, 29-31		

By far the most famous descendent of David was Jesus. In the New Testament Jesus is referred to the "son of David" in many passages of scripture. Both Mary, His mother, and Joseph, His adopted father, traced their lineage to King David (Matthew 1, Luke 3). What did Paul say in Romans 1:2-4 about Jesus' heritage?

_____

_____

_____

But David's legacy to Jesus is more than mere ancestry. What did people say about Jesus as He conducted His ministry? Read Matthew 12:23 for an answer.

_____

_____

_____

The title "Son of David" refers to the *Messiah* prophesied in the Hebrew Bible. God promised David that He would establish a dynasty through his sons and that one of his descendants would rule over His kingdom forever. This promised King of the Davidic covenant was given the title *Messiah*, which means "anointed one" or "chosen one." A person was anointed with oil to signify authority or nobility. David was anointed by Samuel when he was told he would become king of Israel (1 Samuel 16:13). An anointing indicated that the person was set apart for God's purposes. The Greek word that corresponds to Messiah is *Christos*, which is transliterated into "Christ" in English. When New Testament people referred to Jesus as "the Son of David," they were referencing this royal connection. They either believed or were questioning if Jesus was the Messiah, the Christ, the promised forever ruler of God's kingdom (e.g., Matthew 15:22, 20:30).

Jesus called Himself the "Offspring of David" in Revelation 22:16, this week's memory verse. Write it here.

_____

_____

_____

Christians share in this royal lineage. What does John 1:12-13 say about our relationship to God through Jesus?

_____

_____

_____

What does 1 Peter 2:9 say about our royal status?

_____

_____

_____

Through Jesus, the son of David, the Messiah, the Christ, you are royalty! You have been adopted into the royal family of God, and you have all the rights and privileges of the child of the King. And as His children, we can choose to live as royalty, confident in our authority in Christ and conducting ourselves as His ambassadors, loving others as He does. This attitude can apply to our food and exercise choices as well. If I am a child of the King, I recognize my freedom to make healthy choices alongside the responsibility to live as one who is fit for a king, acting righteously in light of all God has done for me. How does this truth impact your thinking about yourself and your relationship to God and others?

_____

_____

_____

Jesus, You are the Offspring of David, Messiah, Wonderful Counselor, Mighty God, Everlasting Father, and Prince of Peace. I am grateful to be a part of Your royal family, and I ask You for help in living my life in such a way that honors You and Your gospel. Amen.

—— DAY 2: VICTORY
Holy Lord, I find my strength and hope in You alone. I come to You now knowing You will fill me with Your Word and empower me through Your Spirit.

Another aspect of David's legacy is victory. He had victory over the giant Goliath, King Saul, military enemies, and political intrigue. He knew that being devoted to God involved battles against His enemies. And he also knew the source of the victory. Moses taught the Israelites this principle before they entered the Promised Land after the Exodus. Look up Deuteronomy 20:3-4 and identify their source of victory.

_____

_____

_____

David expressed this idea in one of his psalms. Find Psalm 108:13 and write it here.

_____

_____

_____

We also are engaged in battles today. Some are against the enemy of God and some are against our own tendencies to sin. The good news is that victory is already ours through Jesus. Read His words in John 16:33 and fill in the blanks.

The good news: "In Me you may have _____."

The bad news: "In this world you will have _____."

The best news: "But take heart! I have _____ the world."

Only a few hours before His disciples saw His arrest that led to His crucifixion, He offered these words of comfort and promised them peace and victory. He guaranteed trouble lay ahead, but the victory was assured. Jesus won the battle over sin and its control over us. How does Peter describe this victory in 1 Peter 2:24?

_____

_____

_____

Although we have won the victory we still must participate in the battle every day. One battle we face is temptation, and for many of us that battle includes the temptation to make unhealthy choices in the areas of food and exercise. When I joined First Place (the original name of First Place for Health) in 1981, one of the first verses I memorized was 1 Corinthians 10:13. It continues to be an important weapon in my battle against temptation. If you know it from memory, write it here. If you do not already know it from memory, look it up and write it here. Make an intentional plan to commit it to memory.

_____

_____

_____

As a First Place for Health leader and member, I see how many people struggle with memorizing scripture. How successful have you been during this study to memorize and recite the verses each week? I was inspired by a member of Carole Lewis's group, Leatrice Roberts, who recites all the memory verses at their victory celebration at the end of every session. I recently did the same thing and found great encouragement that God's Word is hidden in my heart not just on the page of a Bible. I was able to do it with God's help and daily practice. What does Ephesians 6:17 say about the Word of God?

_____

_____

_____

Why do we need God's Word (verse 12)?

_____

_____

_____

The Word of God is not only a weapon in the fight against the enemy. God also uses it in the battles within our own hearts. Read Hebrews 4:12; how does this verse describe God's Word?

_____

_____

_____

We fight daily battles to share in the victory Jesus won for us. What will be the eternal result of this victory? Look up James 1:12 to find our promised reward.

_____

_____

_____

In the power of Jesus we are victorious kings. What is one way you can walk in victory with Jesus this week?

_____

_____

_____

I thank You for the victory I have in Jesus, my Savior forever, Who sought me and bought me with His redeeming blood. Show me the victories You have prepared for me today and help me walk in freedom as Your child. Amen.

—— DAY 3: REDEMPTION

As I enter into Your awesome presence, Father, I am reminded that I am only here because of Jesus's loving sacrifice on my behalf. Thank You for rescuing me through the blood of Christ.

The Bible is a story of redemption. God took many broken lives and corrupt societies and rescued them from utter ruin. It started with the exile of Adam and Eve from Eden's garden and continues to today. David's life is part of that legacy of redemption. God took an unlikely shepherd boy to rule a mighty nation and through his line, He provided rescue to all people through Jesus' sacrificial death and resurrection.

Let's look at one of the Bible's stories of redemption, the story of Ruth. Here's the background: During the time of the judges in Israel, there was a famine. Naomi, her husband, and two sons migrated to Moab to find food. While they were there her sons married Moabite women. But tragedy struck. During the ten years they were in Moab, Naomi's husband and both of her sons died, leaving her in a foreign land with no one to care for her. In the culture of the day, her daughters-in-law would need to remarry as soon as possible to start their own families to support them. Naomi heard that the famine in her homeland was over, so she decided to return. Both of her daughters-in-law, Orpah and Ruth, prepared to go with her. Why do you think that they would do this?

_____

_____

_____

The relationship between the three women was based on a covenant: the covenant of marriage. They became a family when the women married Naomi's sons and were thus committed to care for each other for the rest of their lives. But Naomi gave the women an out. What did she say in Ruth 1:8-9?

_____

_____

_____

At Naomi's insistence Orpah returned home. But what did Ruth tell Naomi in verses 16 and 17?

_____

_____

_____

Without a husband, sons, or grandchildren, Naomi faced poverty and the danger of starvation for the rest of her life. Ruth's promise (or covenant) ensured that she would not be left alone. But there is more: Ruth sacrificed her opportunity to remarry and have a family because she would be caring for Naomi. She basically signed up for the same fate Naomi faced: no one to care for her in her old age. She took Naomi's place, giving up her life for hers. Compounding the seriousness of the situation, Ruth was a widow moving to a foreign country, one that was not fond of her nationality. She would not likely find a husband in Israel but instead face prejudice and persecution. But she went anyway, providing hope to Naomi in her destitute state.

When they returned to Naomi's home, Ruth made good on her promise to care for her. She went to the fields during the harvest season to gather grain for their food. According to Mosaic Law farmers were to leave grain in the corners of their fields or grain that was dropped during the harvest so that the poor and foreigners could collect food (Leviticus 19:9-10, Deuteronomy 24:19-22). This process was a way to support the needy in a time when government support didn't exist. But what did God want His people to remember as a part of this practice? Read Deuteronomy 24:22 for the answer.

_____

_____

_____

The scripture does not specifically say that God was moving behind the scenes, but we can infer that truth. God provided for Ruth by sending her to a field owned by a man who was related to Naomi and her family, a man named Boaz. Eventually, Boaz agreed to marry Ruth but first he had to follow some rules found in the Mosaic Law. Look up Deuteronomy 25:5-6; what did a man have to do if his married brother died without any children?

_____

_____

_____

Part of the reason for this law was to keep the family's land intact as part of the tribal distribution of land described in Joshua. If the dead man had no brothers, the nearest male relative took on the role of kinsman redeemer. In Ruth's situation there was someone more closely related to Naomi than Boaz. But when Boaz talked to this man, he refused to marry Ruth, allowing Boaz to take her as his wife (Ruth 4:9-10). Now through the covenant of marriage, both Ruth and Naomi were rescued from poverty and destitution. What happened in Ruth 4:13-16?

_____

_____

_____

How is this story connected to David (verse 17)?

_____

_____

_____

What does this story mean for us today? When we were without hope, Jesus brought hope to us. We were enslaved in the bondage of sin. He left His home in heaven, came to our world, a foreign land, in a mortal body, and suffered our shame, loss, and despair to free us. We were alone and starving for God and He established a new covenant so we can belong to His forever family. He is the groom and we are His bride, the church. He is our kinsman redeemer, as both Ruth and Boaz exemplified in this amazing story. He makes us fit for a king.

How has God redeemed you? Write a prayer of thanks to Him in response to your redemption story.

_____

_____

_____

I love to proclaim my story of redemption through the blood of the Lamb of God. My shackles are gone and I'm free from the slavery of sin. Thank You, Father, for never giving up on humanity or on me. Amen.

—— DAY 4: SPIRIT LED

Holy Spirit, You are my comforter and teacher. Speak to my heart and show me the deep truths of God's Word.

During David's life he was led by the Spirit of God. At the time of his anointing as king, "the Spirit of the Lord came powerfully upon David" from that day on (1

Samuel 16:13). Although he didn't experience the Spirit's indwelling that Christians do today, he was attuned to the Spirit's leadership and consistently responded in obedience. His legacy includes a model of how to live a Spirit led life. Walking in the Spirit is vital to a life characterized by healthy choices. Without God's help, we are powerless to regularly eat and exercise in beneficial ways.

Read Galatians 5:16-17. What does verse 16 say will happen if we walk by the Spirit?

_____

_____

_____

What is in conflict (verse 17)?

_____

_____

_____

How can we walk in the Spirit? Galatians 5:24-25 helps us understand this. Verse 24 says "we belong to Jesus." That is the reason we are able to crucify our self and our fleshly desires. When temptation comes calling, you can say, "I belong to Jesus, and He wants the best for me. This is not His best so I will resist." Because I belong to Jesus, I don't want to participate in things that are opposed to His gospel and His teachings. We are in an exclusive family that lives by a different standard than the one the world practices.

Being led by God's Spirit means we are dead to self but alive to Him (Romans 6:11). How did Jesus describe this process in John 12:24-26?

_____

_____

_____

At times we may struggle with knowing which way the Spirit is leading us. How do we know if we are following the Holy Spirit? Read each of these verses and list the results of a Spirit-led life.

Acts 1:8

_____

_____

_____

2 Timothy 1:7

_____

_____

_____

Galatians 5:22-23

_____

_____

_____

One way to practice walking in the Spirit is at the grocery store. As you walk down each aisle, it can be tempting to put something in your basket that will be a stumbling block to your healthy food plan. Allow the Holy Spirit to direct you as you choose healthier options. Pray that He will keep you away from the aisles containing food that can sabotage your fitness goals. Another way is to actually walk. As you walk, pray or recite scripture to keep in communication with the Holy Spirit. Finally, when you see yourself producing behaviors that are the opposite of the fruit of the Spirit, spend quiet time in prayer asking the Holy Spirit to give you power to walk with Him and cultivate His fruit in your life.

How will you ensure you are being led by the Spirit this week?

_____

_____

_____

Holy Spirit, You are welcome in my heart and in my walk. I thank You for the power of God that lives in me, allowing me to obey and trust my Father. Keep me walking in the paths that He has set before me for my good and His glory. Amen.

—— DAY 5: TOTAL DEVOTION

Father God, I want to have a heart like Yours, one that bends easily to Your will and passionately craves You above all else. Work in me to bring out my best for Your glory.

Of all the things we've studied about David, perhaps the greatest is a legacy of devotion. He had one of the deepest desires to follow God and keep His commands among those whose lives are recorded in scripture. His heart beat to the rhythm of God's Word. He was all in. How can we follow in his footsteps in the area of devotion to God? Read Deuteronomy 17:18-19. This passage comes from Moses' directions for future kings of Israel. What do these verses say the king should do?

_____

_____

_____

Samuel, the judge and prophet who anointed David, gave advice during his last speech to the Israelites. Look up 1 Samuel 12:24; what did he say?

_____

_____

_____

God's Word is our foundation for devotion to Him. Being saturated in His Word results in obedience that is joyful rather than reluctant, eager rather than resistant, and humble rather than proud. David modeled that kind of devotion for us, and Jesus provided teaching and example as well. Jesus gave us a measurement for devotion in relation to food. What did He tell His disciples in John 4:34?

_____

_____

_____

Paul gave us good advice about devotion to God in Romans 12:1-2. What are we to offer to God?

_____

_____

_____

Why?

_____

_____

_____

To what should we not conform?

_____

_____

_____

What should we do instead?

_____
_____
_____

What will be the result?

_____
_____
_____

Find 2 Corinthians 5:14-15. What compels us to live a life devoted to God?

_____
_____
_____

Why are we compelled?

_____
_____
_____

What did Christ do for us (verse 15)?

_____
_____
_____

How should we live in response to what He did?

_____
_____
_____

Based on what you have studied about David and these verses from today's lesson, what does a life totally devoted to God look like in your opinion?

_____
_____
_____

Is anything hindering your total devotion to God in this season of your life? If so, what?

He was a young boy when foreign invaders destroyed his home and took him into slavery in their land. During his captivity his faith in God grew greatly. After six years of hard work and near starvation, he miraculously escaped and made it back home to his family. But he felt an urgent call that would not leave him alone. His heart was drawn back to the land where he had lived in chains. God wanted him to bring the gospel to the same people who had treated him cruelly. The former slave returned to the foreign soil to share the love of Christ. He was in constant danger of the dungeon and death but he pressed on, living in poverty to bring the riches of God to others. After his death he was canonized as a saint, St. Patrick, the patron saint of Ireland. His life is another example of one completely devoted to God and His gospel, regardless of personal cost or challenges. God calls each of us to live a life devoted to Him, completely submitted to His will and His Word. This is what it means to be fit for a king.

I lay my heart before Your throne, dear Lord, and give it all to You. Help me walk each day fully devoted to You, obeying Your Word and loving others as You love them. You have done great things for me; help me to do great things for You. Amen.

—— DAY 6: REFLECTION AND APPLICATION
What joy I find in Your presence, Lord! You are everything I need, and all my heart desires is to know You more. Thank You for Your unending grace and mercy.

Practice reciting this week's memory verse by writing it here.

What does it mean to leave a godly legacy? An example is Susanna Wesley. She had nineteen children and lived a life devoted to God before them. She made sure that she spent at least an hour alone with each child each week and she ensured each one had a sound education. She managed her home with amazing organizational skill. When her pastor husband was away, she would keep the parish running. She had prayer meetings in her home. She helped to originate the idea of lay leaders in the church. Two of her sons, Charles and John, became spiritual leaders whose preaching and writing began the movement that became the Methodist church.[1] They also wrote thousands of hymns, some of which we still sing today such as "O For a Thousand Tongues to Sing." John Wesley said, "I learned more about Christianity from my mother than from all the theologians in England." Susanna Wesley left a legacy that impacted countless numbers of people and continues to reach people for Christ today.

David's legacy has influenced people for thousands of years. His devotion to God, his stories, and his psalms inspire us to develop a heart like God's. What will you leave behind and how will your life represent the God you love? Your legacy is important, not for the number of people you touch but how you touch people.

Being fit for a king—a person who has a heart like God's—involves love that obeys without question. How did King Saul lose the crown? Read 1 Samuel 13:14 for an answer.

_____

_____

_____

David, on the other hand, was committed to obeying God consistently. He was not perfect; none of us is. But God saw in him a heart that was fit for a king, a king who would serve Him and lead His people with integrity. In Psalm 61:6 (TPT) David tells God, "You treat me like a king." Read verse 7 in any translation you wish. What does he ask God to do for him?

_____

_____

_____

What will David do in response (verse 8)?

_____

_____

_____

God wants to treat you like a king. What would you ask God to do for you?

_____

_____

_____

What will you do in response to His answer to your request?

_____

_____

_____

Look back at the topic for each of the previous week's lessons in this study. Here is a list for easy reference.

- David's Calling
- David's Faith
- David's Worship
- David's Songs
- David's Integrity
- David's Rebellion
- David's Humility

Which of these characteristics best represent the legacy you are developing? Why?

_____

_____

_____

Which one of these characteristics would you like to develop more deeply? How?

_____

_____

_____

At the end of the book of 2 Samuel we see the end of David's life. He had some final words for the people. These final words begin with this introduction: "The inspired utterance of David son of Jesse, the utterance of the man exalted by the Most High, the man anointed by the God of Jacob, *the hero of Israel's songs*" (2 Samuel 23:1, emphasis added). David was a hero for many reasons, but in this passage the people remembered him for his songs and his inspiration to follow God and praise and talk with Him constantly. It's a legacy that gives us hope when giants confront us and kings seek to kill us. It's a legacy that calls us to repentance when we sin. It's a legacy that pulls us to our knees in humility before a mighty God. It's a legacy of a king who served his King well.

What will be your legacy? How will your life inspire others to seek God first and love Him with their whole beings? How will your fitness journey show others the way to God's healthy lifestyle in emotion, spirit, mind, and body? Each day you follow God adds to your legacy, and I pray that you will find Him in each moment. His love for you is vast and His plan for you is to be fit for a king.

Expand the days of my life, Lord, that I may dwell in Your presence forever. I will praise You for as long as I live, and I ask that my life be a legacy for You. May everything I do be for Your glory and everything I am be fit for a king, my loving Lord and Father. Amen.

—— DAY 7: REFLECTION AND APPLICATION

My life is in Your hands, Father. I bow before You, knowing that my strength is small but that Yours is mighty. Show me more of You so that I may follow You more closely.

What have you learned during this study? How has God spoken to you about being fit for a king? Take time today to consider your legacy of devotion to God and what He is calling you to do for His Kingdom's work. Here are some prompts that you might use in your meditation or journaling.

- **Create a victory banner.** It can be any shape you chose; one would be a pennant like those used in sports. On your banner write a scripture or phrase that represents the victory you have in Jesus. One example from the Day 1 lesson is John 16:33: "I have overcome the world! –Jesus."
- **Describe a time in your life when you were led by the Spirit** in a direction that was unexpected. How did you know what God wanted you to do? What were the results of your obedience to the Spirit's leadership?
- **Take several slips of paper and on each one write a sin or a selfish desire** that is hard for you to resist. Draw or attach an image of a cross on a journal page. Attach each of the slips of paper to the cross. Write a prayer thanking God that you have crucified your desires and can leave them behind as you walk forward in the Spirit.
- **Write the word devotion in a vertical column** on the left side of your journal page. Beside each letter write a word or phrase that represents devotion. You can include scripture verses as well. For example, for the letter "D" you might write "doing God's will instead of mine."
- **Find a song that encourages you** in this process. You may document the lyrics and record your own reflections on them, or you could illustrate them with sketches or images you locate. Two examples for this week's study are "Legacy" by Nicole Nordeman (2002) and "Only Jesus" by Casting Crowns (2018).

Your journal holds a very private and personal process; therefore, share it carefully. If social media is a healthy place for you, use these hashtags for posting your words, images, other reflections, or personal stories from this study: #fp4h and #fp4hfit-foraking. You can view my journal and others' entries using these hashtags.

Thank You for this session of First Place for Health and for all the ways You have changed me. I appreciate all the members and the leader of my group, and I pray we will continue to seek You and Your Kingdom's better way above all things as we strive to live healthier lives. Without You we are nothing, Lord. But with You we have the victory through Jesus Christ our Lord. I love You. Amen.

_____
_____
_____
_____
_____
_____
_____
_____
_____
_____
_____
_____
_____
_____
_____
_____
_____
_____
_____
_____
_____

1 Acts 2. Step Bible (2023), https://www.stepbible.org/?q=version=ESV|reference=Acts.2&options=HNVUG.
2 John Piper, "Following Christ Is Costly—But How Do You Count the Cost?" Desiring God (2018), https://www.desiringgod.org/interviews/following-christ-is-costly-but-how-do-you-count-the-cost.
3 Oswald Chambers, "Total Surrender," My Utmost for His Highest (2023), https://utmost.org/total-surrender/.

WEEK NINE: A TIME TO CELEBRATE

This study has provided opportunities to learn lessons from the life of David and how to be fit for a king. To help you shape your short victory celebration testimony, work through the following questions in your prayer journal, one on each day leading up to your group's celebration.

DAY ONE: List some of the benefits you have gained by allowing the Lord to transform your life through this First Place for Health session. Be mindful that He has been active in all four aspects of your being, so list benefits you have received in the physical, mental, emotional and spiritual realms.

DAY TWO: In what ways have you most significantly changed mentally? Have you seen a shift in the ways you think about yourself, food, your relationships, or God? How has Scripture memory been a part of these shifts?

DAY THREE: In what ways have you most significantly changed emotionally? Have you begun to identify how your feelings influence your relationship to food and exercise? What are you doing to stay aware of your emotions, both positive and negative?

DAY FOUR: In what ways have you most significantly changed spiritually? How has your relationship with God deepened? How has drawing closer to Him made a difference in the other three areas of your life?

DAY FIVE: In what ways have you most significantly changed physically? Have you met or exceeded your weight/measurement goals? How has your health improved during the past nine weeks?

DAY SIX: Was there one person in your First Place for Health group who was particularly encouraging to you? How did their kindness make a difference in your First Place for Health journey?

DAY SEVEN: Summarize the previous six questions into a one-page testimony, or "faith story," to share at your group's victory celebration.

As you live out your life as one who is fit for a king, continue to put Christ first in all things and love Him with your whole being in all things!

LEADER DISCUSSION GUIDE

For in-depth information, guidance, and helpful tips about leading a successful First Place for Health group, spend time studying the *My Place for Leadership* book. In it, you will find valuable answers to most of your questions, as well as personal insights from many First Place for Health group leaders.

For the group meetings in this session, be sure to read and consider each week's discussion topics several days before the meeting—some questions and activities require supplies and/or planning to complete. Also, if you are leading a large group, plan to break into smaller groups for discussion and then come together as a large group to share your answers and responses. Make sure to appoint a capable leader for each small group so that discussions stay focused and on track (and be sure each group records their answers!).

——WEEK ONE: DAVID'S CALLING

1. As you begin the first lesson of this session, encourage your members to participate and ask questions during each week's discussion. You may start with an open-ended question such as, "What do you think the title of this Bible study tells us about what we will be studying?"
2. Ask members to identify a person in the Bible who is their favorite one to study and explain why.
3. Review the Week 1 summary at the beginning of the Week 2 lesson. Ask members to think about what they learned about David's calling to be king.
4. Lead a discussion about how outward appearances can often be deceiving.
5. Identify the lessons about being a shepherd in Day 2. Ask members how God fulfills these roles in their lives.
6. Ask members to discuss how music affects them in their relationship to God.
7. Review the story about Tanya Murphy in the Day 6 lesson. Ask for volunteers to share how God has called them into a ministry or service that stems from a situation in their lives.
8. Encourage members to share any reflections or journaling they did during the week if they feel comfortable doing so. You might split the group up into pairs or small groups for journal and reflection sharing.
9. End the meeting by leading the group in reading aloud the prayer from Day 7, with each member putting her name in the blanks.

——WEEK TWO: DAVID'S FAITH

1. Review the Week 2 summary at the beginning of the Week 3 lesson. Ask members to think about what they learned about David's faith.

2. Go over the three obstacles David faced that are discussed in Day 1. Ask members to share a time when they faced any of these obstacles in a difficult situation and how they trusted in God for victory.

3. Lead a discussion about David's faith in battle from Day 2. Why do you think faith in God may be easier or harder when you face a difficult circumstance?

4. Read this quote from Day 3 and ask volunteers to comment on it: "If we focus on trusting God, He will take care of the rest. It doesn't mean things will be easy, but expending our energy on pursuing God rather than leaning on our own understanding and strength is much easier in the long run."

5. Talk about a friend who has been an important part of your life. Ask other members to share about their friendships.

6. Ask members to share their thoughts about Gideon and Barak's questioning faith and how they are worthy to be in the Hebrews 11 Hall of Faith.

7. Encourage members to share any reflections or journaling they did during the week if they feel comfortable doing so. You might split the group up into pairs or small groups for journal and reflection sharing.

—— WEEK THREE: DAVID'S WORSHIP

1. Review the Week 3 summary at the beginning of the Week 4 lesson. Ask members to think about what they learned about David's worship.

2. Lead a discussion about what worship means to your group members. What does worshipping with abandon look like for them?

3. Ask members how they practice God's presence during corporate worship and during the rest of the week. How does God's presence fit into your everyday activities?

4. What does prayer look like for you and your members? Talk about the successes and challenges of praying as a part of worship.

5. Read the story from Philip Yancey at the beginning of Day 4. Call on volunteers who want to share similar stories of experiencing deep reverence for God.

6. Ask members to talk about how God fills them in ways that nothing else does. Does the urge to eat signal that they are hungry for something else? If so, what?

7. Encourage members to share any reflections or journaling they did during the week if they feel comfortable doing so. You might split the group up into pairs or small groups for journal and reflection sharing.

—— WEEK FOUR: DAVID'S SONGS

1. Review the Week 4 summary at the beginning of the Week 5 lesson. Ask members to think about what they learned about David's songs.

2. Ask members to share their favorite psalm and why it is their favorite.

3. Call on a volunteer to read Psalm 103 aloud. What aspects of praise do you notice in this psalm?

4. Review the three songs described in Day 2. You can choose one to play and invite group members to sing along.

5. Share your prayer of lament that you wrote for Day 3. Ask other members to share their prayers. Why is lament an important part of David's songs?

6. Lead a discussion about petition in prayer. How do you pray for yourself and others, and how do you see God responding to your petitions?

7. Read this quote from Day 5: "The power of gratitude can change long hours of waiting to mere minutes. It is more powerful than any situation." Ask members to comment on this quote about gratitude and share any personal stories about how God has used gratitude to change their perspective.

8. Encourage members to share any reflections or journaling they did during the week if they feel comfortable doing so. You might split the group up into pairs or small groups for journal and reflection sharing.

—— WEEK FIVE: DAVID'S INTEGRITY

1. Review the Week 5 summary at the beginning of the Week 6 lesson. Ask members to think about what they learned about David's integrity.

2. David started his reign as king dedicated to integrity. Ask members to describe a time when they started something new with a goal of staying devoted to God or remaining true to His ways. This can include starting a new First Place for Health session.

3. Lead a discussion about the relationship between leaders and their followers. What does a leader with integrity look like?

4. David waited a long time to become king. Ask members to talk about how waiting can prepare you for a position of leadership. How hard is it to wait and still act with consistent integrity?

5. Ask members to talk about a time when they were in crisis and faced a decision that could compromise their integrity. How did they handle the situation and what part did God play in it?

6. Pose this question: If auditors looked at your financial records, how would they know that you are a follower of Jesus?

7. Talk to your members about lifelong fitness as a goal rather than just losing weight for a session of First Place for Health. What are the differences between those two mindsets?

8. Encourage members to share any reflections or journaling they did during the week if they feel comfortable doing so. You might split the group up into pairs or small groups for journal and reflection sharing.

—— WEEK SIX: DAVID'S REBELLION

1. Review the Week 6 summary at the beginning of the Week 7 lesson. Ask members to think about what they learned about David's rebellion.
2. Trace the steps David took to his sins of adultery and murder. Ask members how we can we avoid temptation and rebellion.
3. Discuss the importance of accountability in our spiritual and fitness journey. How could an accountability partner have helped David after he sinned?
4. Ask members to talk about David's family problems due to his multiple marriages.
5. Review David's rebellion with the census. How did pride influence him to sin?
6. David was passive in many of his relationships. How did that cause problems and how could he have prevented them?
7. Read this quote and ask for volunteers to comment on it: "There is hope for us when we don't obey God, and we can be restored to a right relationship with Him no matter what we have done. When we make unhealthy choices with food, it is not the end of our story."
8. Encourage members to share any reflections or journaling they did during the week if they feel comfortable doing so. You might split the group up into pairs or small groups for journal and reflection sharing.

—— WEEK SEVEN: DAVID'S HUMILITY

1. Review the Week 7 summary at the beginning of the Week 8 lesson. Ask members to think about what they learned about David's humility.
2. Call on each member and ask them to share one thing for which they are thankful. How does being thankful to God develop humility?
3. Ask members how they respond to their own sins and failures. Do they go to God immediately and ask forgiveness or do they avoid facing the truth? Why is humility so important in receiving forgiveness?
4. Discuss accepting difficult situations and how God can give us peace in the storms of life. How has God walked alongside you in a difficult time?
5. Ask a member to read Philippians 2:5-8. What does Jesus' example of humble servanthood mean to you? How do you follow His example?
6. Pose this question: If you were to choose one word to be engraved on your tombstone, what would it be and why?
7. Lead a discussion about the difficulties of obedience. Why do we resist being obedient to God when we know it is always best for us?
8. Encourage members to share any reflections or journaling they did during the week if they feel comfortable doing so. You might split the group up into pairs or small groups for journal and reflection sharing.

—— WEEK EIGHT: DAVID'S LEGACY

1. Share this summary for Week Eight. Ask members to think about what they learned about David's legacy.

    - David's royal line culminated in Jesus, the prophesied King of Kings, who makes us fit to be kings as God's adopted children.
    - God's Word is a vital weapon in our victory over the enemy and our fleshly desires so we should commit as much of it to memory as we can.
    - The Bible is a story of redemption, God rescuing us from the curse of sin and death and giving us a place in His family forever.
    - Walking in the Spirit includes living by God's leadership rather than following the world's ways or personal preferences.
    - Devotion to God means our hearts beat to the rhythm of God's Word.

2. Ask members to share what legacies they want to leave after they are gone. What steps are important to leaving these legacies?

3. David was an ancestor of Jesus, the Messiah promised throughout the Old Testament. Ask members to share connections between David and Jesus they saw in the Day 1 lesson or that they already knew.

4. Review John 16:33. Lead a discussion about the victory we experience in Jesus through His death and resurrection.

5. Trace the story of Ruth, Naomi, and Boaz. How does this story help us understand God's redemptive mission?

6. Lead a discussion about practical ways to walk in the Spirit such as walking through the grocery store as described in Day 4.

7. Call on a member to read 2 Corinthians 5:14-15 to the group. What does it look like to be compelled to live for Christ and not ourselves? How will this lifestyle affect the legacies we leave?

8. Review the weekly topics listed in Day 6 and ask members to share their responses to the questions regarding them.

9. Encourage members to share any reflections or journaling they did during the week if they feel comfortable doing so. You might split the group up into pairs or small groups for journal and reflection sharing.

—— WEEK NINE: TIME TO CELEBRATE

As your class members reflect the weekly content of *Fit for a King*, help them remember the lessons they have learned from David's life. Ask them what they have learned about David's characteristics and how God is developing those character traits in them.

FIRST PLACE FOR HEALTH
JUMP START MENUS

All recipe and menu nutritional information was determined using the Master-Cook software, a program that accesses a database containing more than 6,000 food items prepared using the United States Department of Agriculture (USDA) publications and information from food manufacturers.

As with any nutritional program, MasterCook calculates the nutritional values of the recipes based on ingredients. Nutrition may vary due to how the food is prepared, where the food comes from, soil content, season, ripeness, processing and method of preparation. You are expected to add snacks and sides as needed to meet your nutritional needs. For these reasons, please use the recipes and menu plans as approximate guides. As always, consult your physician and/or a registered dietitian before starting a weight-loss program.

Apple-Cinnamon Quinoa Bowl

¾ cup low-fat milk
⅔ cup diced apple, divided
¼ cup quinoa
¼ teaspoon ground cinnamon
⅛ teaspoon salt
4 teaspoons sliced almonds
½ teaspoon honey

Combine milk, 1/3 cup apple, quinoa, cinnamon and salt in a small saucepan. Bring to a boil. Cover and simmer on very low heat until the liquid is absorbed, about 12 minutes. Serves 1

Let stand 5 minutes. Top with the remaining 1/3 cup apple, almonds and honey.

Nutritional Information: 331 Calories, 8g Fat, 9mg Cholesterol, 52g Carbohydrate, 6g Fiber, 374mg Sodium

Stuffed Sweet Potato with Hummus Dressing

1 large sweet potato, scrubbed
¾ cup chopped kale
1 cup canned black beans, rinsed
¼ cup hummus
2 tablespoons water

Prick sweet potato all over with a fork. Microwave on High until cooked through.

Meanwhile, wash kale and drain, allowing water to cling to the leaves. Place in a medium saucepan; cover and cook over medium-high heat, stirring once or twice, until wilted. Add beans; add a tablespoon or two of water if the pot is dry. Continue cooking, uncovered, stirring occasionally, until the mixture is steaming hot, 1 to 2 minutes.

Split the sweet potato open and top with the kale and bean mixture. Combine hummus and 2 tablespoons water in a small dish. Add additional water as needed to reach desired consistency. Drizzle the hummus dressing over the stuffed sweet potato. Serves 1

Nutritional Information: 472 Calories, 7g Fat, 85g Carbohydrate, 21g Protein, 22g Fiber, 489mg Sodium

BBQ Chicken Breasts with Apricot

4 chicken breast halves (about 1 1/2 lbs.) skin on and bone in

1/3 cup apricot preserves

1 tablespoon soy sauce

1 tablespoon water

2 tablespoon plus 2 teaspoon ketchup

2 teaspoon brown sugar

Preheat grill to medium. Grill chicken (skin on) 10 minutes, turning occasionally. Remove from grill and remove skin. In small bowl, combine preserves, soy sauce, water, ketchup and brown sugar, blend well. Return chicken to grill, generously brush with glaze. Continue cooking 10 to 15 minutes or until thoroughly done, turning often and brushing with glaze frequently. Serves 4.

Nutritional Information: 515 Calories, 17g Fat, 91mg Cholesterol, 56g Carbohydrate, 35g Protein, 8g Fiber, 941mg Sodium

DAY 2 | BREAKFAST

Blueberry Smoothie

1½ cups frozen blueberries
1¼ cups almond milk, plus more as needed
1 cup frozen cauliflower
½ cup frozen raspberries
½ frozen banana
2 tablespoons almond butter
1 tablespoon maple syrup
1 tablespoon fresh lemon juice

In a blender, place the blueberries, almond milk, cauliflower, raspberries, banana, almond butter, maple syrup, and lemon juice.

Blend until creamy, adding more almond milk as needed to blend. Serves 3

Nutritional Informational: 322 Calories, 7g Fat, 3mg Cholesterol, 62g Carohydrate, 6g Protein, 7g Fiber, 38mg Sodium

Chickpea & Veggie Grain Bowl

1 cup cooked quinoa
1 cup mixed salad greens
1 cup roasted root vegetables
¼ cup canned chickpeas, rinsed
1 tablespoon crumbled feta cheese

Combine quinoa, greens, roasted vegetables, chickpeas and feta in a bowl. Serves 1

Nutritional Information: 303 Calories, 10g Fat, 44g Carbohydrate, 9g Fiber, 20g Protein, 8mg Cholesterol, 387mg Sodium

Chicken Cacciatore Pie

1 lb. ground chicken breast
1 15-ounce can Italian-style diced tomatoes, drained (reserve 3 1/2 table-spoon juice)
3/4 small onion, chopped
3/4 small green bell pepper, chopped
1 garlic clove, minced
1/3 cup plain bread crumbs
1 egg
1 1/4 teaspoon Italian herb seasoning
1/3 cup fat-free mozzarella cheese, shredded
2 tablespoon Parmesan cheese, grated

Preheat oven to 350°F. In medium bowl, combine reserved tomato juice, onion, bell pepper, garlic, bread crumbs and egg. Add half the Italian seasoning, salt and pepper to taste. Mix thoroughly. Add ground chicken, mix well. Pat mixture evenly into lightly oiled 10-inch pie plate, pushing up sides to form a shell. Bake 25 minutes. In stainless steel saucepan, combine tomatoes and remaining Italian seasoning, salt and pepper to taste. Simmer 10 to 15 minutes over medium heat, remove from heat and set aside. Remove meat shell from oven, discard excess liquid. Sprinkle shell with mozzarella cheese. Add tomato sauce, sprinkle with Parmesan cheese and bake 15 minutes until meat shell is cooked throughout. Let stand 5 minutes before cutting and serving. Serves 4.

Nutritional Information: 348 Calories; 18g Fat, 12g Protein, 34g Carbohydrate, 5g Dietary Fiber, 57mg Cholesterol, 940mg Sodium

Pumpkin-Oatmeal Muffins

3 ½ cups old-fashioned rolled oats
1 ½ cups reduced-fat milk
1 cup unseasoned pumpkin puree
½ cup light brown sugar
1 ½ teaspoons vanilla extract
1 teaspoon baking powder
1 teaspoon pumpkin pie spice
¾ teaspoon salt
2 large eggs, lightly beaten
½ cup chopped pecans

Preheat oven to 375°F. Stir oats, milk, pumpkin, brown sugar, vanilla, baking powder, pumpkin pie spice, salt and eggs together in a large bowl until fully incorporated. Lightly coat a 12-cup muffin tin with cooking spray. Spoon batter into prepared muffin cups, filling each almost to the top. Sprinkle evenly with pecans. Bake muffins until a toothpick inserted in the center comes out clean, 25 to 30 minutes. Let cool in pan for 10 minutes, then transfer to wire rack. Serve warm or at room temperature. Serves 12

Storing: Wrap tightly and refrigerate for up to 2 days or freeze for up to 3 months.

Nutritional Information: 183 Calories, 6g Fat, 33mg Cholesterol, 28g Carbohydrate, 3g Fiber, 6g Protein, 212mg Sodium

Turkey-Apple-Brie Sandwiches

1 Granny Smith apple, thinly sliced
1 teaspoon lemon juice
1 whole-wheat baguette (8 ounces)
4 leaves red leaf lettuce
1 cup shredded cooked turkey breast
2 ounces Brie cheese, thinly sliced
4 teaspoons Dijon mustard

Toss apple slices and lemon juice in a small bowl. Cut baguette crosswise into 4 sections. Cut each section in half lengthwise. Remove the soft inner portion of bread, leaving a 1/4-inch-thick shell. (Reserve the inner bread for another use.) Top the bottom pieces of bread with lettuce, turkey, Brie and the apple slices. Spread mustard on top pieces and set one on each sandwich. Serve immediately or wrap and refrigerate for up to 4 hours. Serves 4

Tip: To cook turkey, place 1 turkey breast tenderloin in a skillet with 1 cup water. Bring to a boil. Reduce heat, cover and simmer until internal temperature reaches 165 degrees F, 20 to 25 minutes. Remove from pan. When cool enough to handle, shred with 2 forks. Refrigerate any remaining turkey in an airtight container for up to 3 days or freeze for up to 2 months.

Nutritional Information: 236 Calories, 5g Fat, 34mg Cholesterol, 32g Carbohydrate, 17g Protein, 5g Fiber, 431mg Sodium

Pesto Ravioli with Spinach & Tomatoes

2 8-ounce packages frozen or refrigerated cheese ravioli
1 tablespoon olive oil
1 pint grape tomatoes
1 5-ounce package baby spinach
⅓ cup pesto

Bring a large pot of water to a boil. Cook ravioli according to package directions; drain and set aside. Heat oil in a large nonstick skillet over medium heat. Add tomatoes; sauté until they begin to burst, 3 to 4 minutes. Add spinach and continue to cook, stirring frequently, until it wilts, 1 to 2 minutes. Add the cooked ravioli and pesto; stir gently to combine.

Nutrition Facts: 361 Calories, 19g Fat, 35g Carbohydrates, 14g Protein

DAY 4 | BREAKFAST

Mini Banana Cake

1/2 cup all-purpose flour
1/2 cup whole-wheat flour
1/2 teaspoon baking powder
1/4 teaspoon baking soda
1/4 teaspoon ground cinnamon
1/8 teaspoon salt
1 1/4 cups buttermilk, at room temperature
1/4 cup unsalted butter, melted and cooled
1 tablespoon light brown sugar plus 1/4 cup, divided
1 teaspoon vanilla extract
2 small bananas, sliced 1/3-inch thick (24 slices)

Preheat oven to 400°F. Coat a 24-cup mini-muffin tray with cooking spray. Whisk all-purpose flour, whole-wheat flour, baking powder, baking soda, cinnamon and salt together in a medium bowl. Whisk buttermilk, butter, 1 tablespoon brown sugar and vanilla in a medium bowl until combined. Gently fold the buttermilk mixture into the flour mixture until just combined. Divide the remaining 1/4 cup brown sugar among the prepared muffin cups (1/2 teaspoon each). Place 1 banana slice atop the sugar in each cup. Spoon batter evenly over each banana slice, about 1 heaping tablespoon per cup. Bake until lightly browned and a wooden pick inserted in the center comes out clean, 10 to 12 minutes. Let cool in the pan for 5 minutes. Run a spatula around the edges to loosen, then gently turn the pan upside down to remove the cakes. Transfer to a platter, banana-side up. Serves 8

Storing: Refrigerate cooled cakes in an airtight container for up to 3 days.

Nutritional Information: 170 Calories, 26g Carbohydrates, 2g Fiber 3g Protein, 17mg Cholesterol, 178mg Sodium

Asiago and Asparagus Omelet

3 stalks asparagus
2 eggs
2 tablespoons water
Salt and fresh ground pepper to taste
1 ounce sliced Asiago cheese

Chop the asparagus stalks, leaving the tops for garnish. Steam the chopped stalks until tender (about 4 to 8 minutes). Heat nonstick pan that has been brushed with oil. Whisk together eggs, water, salt, and pepper. Pour egg mixture into pan, swirling around and lifting gently so that all eggs cook. While eggs are cooking, place the steamed asparagus and cheese on half of the omelet. Gently fold the other half over. Once set, lift and move omelet to serve or keep in warm oven until all omelets are ready. Arrange reserved asparagus around omelet. Serves 1.

Nutritional Information: 292 Calories, 18g Fat, 449mg Cholesterol, 12g Carbohydrate, 21g Protein, 1g Fiber, 489mg Sodium

Seared Salmon with Green Beans

2 Tbsp. plus 2 tsp. olive oil, divided
1 1/4 lb. skinless salmon fillet, cut into 4 portions
1 lb. green beans, trimmed
Kosher salt and pepper
4 cloves garlic, smashed and thinly sliced
1 small red chile, thinly sliced
2 Tbsp. capers, drained, patted dry
Lemon wedges, for serving

Heat 2 teaspoons oil in a large skillet on medium-high. Season salmon with ½ teaspoon each salt and pepper, add to skillet, flesh side down, reduce heat to medium, and cook until golden brown and just opaque throughout, 5 to 6 minutes per side. Remove salmon. Heat remaining 2 tablespoons oil in a large skillet on medium-high. Add green beans and cook until browned, 2½ minutes. Turn and cook until browned and just barely tender, about 3 minutes more.

Remove from heat and toss with ¼ teaspoon salt, then garlic, chile, and capers. Return to medium heat and cook, tossing until garlic is golden brown, 1 to 2 minutes. Serve with salmon and lemon wedges if desired. Serves 4

Nutritional Information (per serving): 285 Calories, 14.5g Fat, 31g Protein, 9g Carbohydrate, 3g Fiber, 540mg Sodium

Yogurt Toast

2 thick slices of bread such as brioche, wheat or sourdough
1/4 cup Greek yogurt
1 large egg
2 Tbsp. maple syrup
Pinch of cinnamon
Blueberries, strawberries, and/or raspberries, for topping
Powdered sugar, toasted oats, dried coconut, chocolate shavings (all optional), for serving

Preheat oven to 400°F. In a medium bowl, whisk yogurt, egg, maple syrup, and cinnamon. Using your fingers or the back of a spoon, press into the center of the bread to indent and create a well. Fill with custard mixture, dividing evenly between the slices. Top the custard with your berry (or mix of berries) of choice. Place prepared bread slices on a baking sheet and bake until the custard is set and the bread is golden brown, 10 to 13 minutes. Transfer to a plate and drizzle lightly with more syrup and optionally finish with a dusting of powdered sugar. Serves 1

Nutritional Information: 348 Calories, 2.2g Fat, 1mg Cholesterol, 57g Carbohydrate, 6g Fiber, 562mg Sodium

DAY 5 | LUNCH

Creamy Pasta Salad

3 cups cooked rotini pasta
1 cup broccoli florets
1 cup quartered cherry tomatoes
3/4 cup diced lean ham (3 ounces)
1/2 cup sliced carrot
1/2 cup sliced red onion
1/3 cup sliced ripe olives
1/4 cup grated Parmesan cheese
2 tablespoons chopped fresh or 2 teaspoons dried basil
2 tablespoons chopped fresh parsley or 2 teaspoons dried parsley flakes
1/4 cup fat-free sour cream
1/4 cup low-fat buttermilk
1/4 cup light ranch dressing

Combine first 10 ingredients in a bowl. Combine sour cream, buttermilk, and dressing; stir well. Pour over salad; toss to coat. Serves 4.

Nutritional Information: 296 Calories, 5g Fat, 12mg Cholesterol, 48g Carbohydrate, 13g Protein, 3g Fiber, 597mg Sodium

BBQ Chicken Tacos with Red Cabbage Slaw

⅓ cup nonfat plain Greek yogurt
1 tablespoon sugar
1 tablespoon lemon juice
1 tablespoon cider vinegar
¾ teaspoon kosher salt
¼ teaspoon ground pepper
Dash of hot sauce
2 cups shredded red cabbage (1/2 head)
2 cups shredded cooked chicken breast (about 6 oz.)
⅓ cup light barbecue sauce
8 corn tortillas
Chopped cilantro for garnish

Combine yogurt, sugar, lemon juice, vinegar, salt, pepper and hot sauce in a large bowl. Add cabbage and toss until fully coated.

Combine chicken and barbecue sauce in a medium microwaveable bowl; toss until the chicken is coated. Microwave on High until heated through, about 1 minute.

Heat tortillas according to package directions. Fill each tortilla with 1/4 cup of the chicken and top with 3 tablespoons of the slaw. Garnish with cilantro and serve. Serves 4

Nutritional Information: 275 Calories, 4g Fat, 60mg Cholesterol, 31g Carbohydrate, 3g Fiber, 26g Protein, 662mg Sodium

Easy Breakfast Tostadas

8 100% corn tortillas

1 tablespoon extra-virgin olive oil

2 cups refried beans, warmed

½ cup grated low-fat sharp cheddar cheese

8 eggs, scrambled

2 cups pico de gallo

To prepare the crispy tortillas: Preheat the oven to 400°F with two racks placed near the middle of the oven. Line two large rimmed baking sheets with parchment paper for easy cleanup. Place tortillas in one layer on baking sheets, brush both sides of each tortilla lightly with oil. Bake for 10 to 12 minutes, turning halfway, until each tortilla is golden and lightly crisp. Set aside. Meanwhile, prepare the remaining components (refried beans, pico de gallo, and preferred eggs). To assemble, spread warm refried beans over each tostada. Top with a sprinkle of cheese, cooked egg and top with pico de gallo. Top with any optional garnishes you'd like, and serve promptly. Serves 8

Nutritional Information per Tostada: 427 Calories, 28g Fat, 379 Cholesterol, 25g Carbohydrate, 17g Protein, 3g Fiber, 549mg Sodium

Grilled Goat Cheese Sandwich

2 teaspoons honey
1/4 teaspoon grated lemon rind
1 4-ounce package goat cheese
8 1-ounce slices cinnamon-raisin bread
2 tablespoons fig preserves
2 teaspoons thinly sliced fresh basil
Cooking spray
1 teaspoon powdered sugar

Combine first 3 ingredients, stirring until well blended. Spread 1 tablespoon goat cheese mixture on each of 4 bread slices; top each slice with 1 1/2 teaspoons preserves and 1/2 teaspoon basil. Top with remaining bread slices. Lightly coat outside of bread with cooking spray. Heat a large nonstick skillet over medium heat. Add 2 sandwiches to pan. Place a cast-iron or heavy skillet on top of sandwiches; press gently to flatten. Cook 3 minutes on each side or until bread is lightly toasted (leave cast-iron skillet on sandwiches while they cook). Repeat with remaining sandwiches. Sprinkle with sugar.

Nutritional Information: 288 Calories, 11g Fat, 13g Protein, 30mg Cholesterol, 34g Carbohydrate, 2g Fiber, 240mg Sodium

Sheet-Pan Parmesan Chicken & Vegetables

4 cups broccoli florets
3 cups cauliflower florets
1 cup sliced shallots
3 tablespoons extra-virgin olive oil, divided
½ teaspoon salt, divided
½ teaspoon ground pepper, divided
2 large cloves garlic, minced
1 teaspoon dried marjoram
4 large bone-in chicken thighs, skin removed if desired
3 tablespoons balsamic vinegar
⅓ cup grated Parmesan cheese

Preheat oven to 450°F. Coat a large rimmed baking sheet with cooking spray. Combine broccoli, cauliflower, shallots, 2 tablespoons oil, 1/4 teaspoon salt and 1/4 teaspoon pepper in a large bowl. Toss well to coat. Transfer to the prepared baking sheet. Combine garlic, marjoram and the remaining 1 tablespoon oil and 1/4 teaspoon each salt and pepper in a small bowl. Coat both sides of the chicken with the garlic mixture. Place on the baking sheet. Roast the chicken and vegetables for 15 minutes. Toss the vegetables and drizzle the chicken with vinegar. Sprinkle all with Parmesan and continue roasting until the vegetables are tender and an instant-read thermometer inserted in the thickest part of the chicken without touching bone registers 165°F, about 10 more minutes. Serves 4

Nutritional Information: 408 Calories, 22g Fat, 160mg Cholesterol, 18g Carbohydrate, 36g Protein, 5g Fiber, 585mg Sodium

Applesauce Muffins

2 cups whole wheat flour
2/3 cup old-fashioned whole rolled oats
1 teaspoon ground cinnamon
3/4 teaspoon baking soda
1 teaspoon baking powder
1/2 teaspoon salt
1 1/3 cups unsweetened applesauce, at room temperature
2 large eggs, at room temperature
1/3 cup coconut oil, melted (or vegetable oil or melted butter)
1/3 cup pure maple syrup, at room temperature
1/3 cup milk (dairy or nondairy), at room temperature
1 teaspoon pure vanilla extract
3/4 cup raisins

Preheat oven to 425°F. Spray a 12-count muffin pan with nonstick spray or use cupcake liners. If using cupcake liners, spray the liners so they won't stick. Whisk the flour, oats, cinnamon, baking soda, baking powder, and salt together in a large bowl until combined. Set aside. In a medium bowl, whisk the applesauce, eggs, oil, maple syrup, milk, and vanilla until combined. Pour the wet ingredients into the dry ingredients and stir. Add the raisins. Fold everything together gently just until combined. Spoon the batter muffin tin, filling them all the way to the top. Top with oats and a light sprinkle of coarse sugar, if desired. Bake for 5 minutes at 425°F. Reduce the oven temperature to 350°F Bake for an additional 15-16 minutes or until a toothpick inserted in the center comes out clean. Cool for 5 minutes in the muffin pan and transfer to a wire rack to continue cooling or enjoy warm. Store in refrigerator for up to one week or in freezer for three months.

Nutritional Information per Muffin: 181 calories, 7.2g fat, 27g carbohydrates, 3.3g fiber, 4g protein, 248mg Sodium

Pita Pizza

2 medium pita breads (about 6 inches)
4 minced garlic cloves
Bunch of fresh basil
2 sliced tomatoes
1/2 cup shredded mozzarella cheese
2 teaspoons extra virgin olive oil

Preheat oven to 400°F. Separate each pita into two. Put pita bread on cookie sheets. Spread 1 minced garlic clove onto each pita round. Arrange 4-6 basil leaves over garlic. Top with 3 slices of tomato. Sprinkle about 2 tablespoons of shredded cheese on each and drizzle with olive oil. Bake for about 15 minutes or until cheese melts and pizzas are bubbly. Serve as whole pizza immediately.

Nutritional Information: 154 Calories, 6g Fat, 6g Protein, 19g Carbohydrate, 1g Dietary Fiber, 13mg Cholesterol, 221mg Sodium

Creamy Broccoli-Cauliflower Chicken Casserole

4 cups cauliflower florets (1-inch)
4 cups broccoli florets (1-inch)
2 tablespoons extra-virgin olive oil
1 cup chopped onion
2 cloves garlic, minced
2 tablespoons all-purpose flour
½ teaspoon salt
½ teaspoon ground pepper
2 cups reduced-fat milk
2 ounces reduced-fat cream cheese, at room temperature
1 cup grated Parmesan cheese, divided
3 cups shredded or chopped cooked chicken

Preheat oven to 375°F. Coat an 8-inch-square baking dish with cooking spray. Bring an inch or two of water to a boil in a large saucepan fitted with a steamer basket. Add cauliflower and broccoli; steam, covered, until almost tender, about 5 minutes. Transfer the vegetables to a rimmed baking sheet and pat dry. Discard the water and wipe out the pot. Heat oil in the saucepan over medium heat. Add onion; cook, stirring, until starting to soften, about 3 minutes. Add garlic; cook, stirring, until fragrant, about 1 minute. Sprinkle with flour, salt and pepper; cook, stirring, for 1 minute. Increase heat to medium-high and whisk in milk and cream cheese. Cook, whisking, until the cream cheese is incorporated and the sauce has thickened, 2 to 3 minutes. Remove from heat and stir in 3/4 cup Parmesan. Add the broccoli, cauliflower and chicken and stir to coat. Transfer to the prepared baking dish. Sprinkle with the remaining 1/4 cup Parmesan. Bake until bubbling around the edges and lightly browned on top, about 20 minutes. Serves 6

Nutritional Information: 327 Calories, 14g Fat, 83mg Cholesterol, 17g Carbohydrate, 32g Protein, 3g Fiber, 594mg Sodium

STEPS FOR SPIRITUAL GROWTH

—— GOD'S WORD FOR YOUR LIFE

I have hidden your word in my heart that I might not sin against you.

Psalm 119:11

As you begin to make decisions based on what God's Word teaches you, you will want to memorize what He has promised to those who trust and follow Him. Second Peter 1:3 tells us that God "has given us everything we need for life and godliness through our knowledge of him" (emphasis added). The Bible provides instruction and encouragement for any area of life in which you may be struggling. If you are dealing with a particular emotion or traumatic life event—fear, discouragement, stress, financial upset, the death of a loved one, a relationship difficulty—you can search through a Bible concordance for Scripture passages that deal with that particular situation. Scripture provides great comfort to those who memorize it.

One of the promises of knowing and obeying God's Word is that it gives you wisdom, insight, and understanding above all worldly knowledge (see Psalm 119:97–104). Psalm 119:129–130 says, "Your statutes are wonderful; therefore I obey them. The unfolding of your words gives light; it gives understanding to the simple." Now that's a precious promise about guidance for life!

The Value of Scripture Memory

Scripture memory is an important part of the Christian life. There are four key reasons to memorize Scripture:

1. **TO HANDLE DIFFICULT SITUATIONS.** A heartfelt knowledge of God's Word will equip you to handle any situation that you might face. Declaring such truth as, "I can do everything through Christ" (see Philippians 4:13) and "he will never leave me or forsake me" (see Hebrews 13:5) will enable you to walk through situations with peace and courage.

2. **TO OVERCOME TEMPTATION.** Luke 4:1–13 describes how Jesus used Scripture to overcome His temptations in the desert (see also Matthew 4:1-11). Knowledge of Scripture and the strength that comes with the ability to use it are important parts of putting on the full armor of God in preparation for spiritual warfare (see Ephesians 6:10–18).

3. **TO GET GUIDANCE.** Psalm 119:105 states the Word of God "is a lamp to my feet and a light for my path." You learn to hide God's Word in your heart so His light will direct your decisions and actions throughout your day.

4. **TO TRANSFORM YOUR MIND.** "Do not conform any longer to the pattern of this world, but be transformed by the renewing of your mind" (Romans 12:2). Scripture memory allows you to replace a lie with the truth of God's Word. When Scripture becomes firmly settled in your memory, not only will your thoughts connect with God's thoughts, but you will also be able to honor God with small everyday decisions as well as big life-impacting ones. Scripture memorization is the key to making a permanent lifestyle change in your thought patterns, which brings balance to every other area of your life.

Scripture Memory Tips

- Write the verse down, saying it aloud as you write it.
- Read verses before and after the memory verse to get its context.
- Read the verse several times, emphasizing a different word each time.
- Connect the Scripture reference to the first few words.
- Locate patterns, phrases, or keywords.
- Apply the Scripture to circumstances you are now experiencing.
- Pray the verse, making it personal to your life and inserting your name as the recipient of the promise or teaching. (Try that with 1 Corinthians 10:13, inserting "me" and "I" for "you.")
- Review the verse every day until it becomes second nature to think those words whenever your circumstances match its message. The Holy Spirit will bring the verse to mind when you need it most if you decide to plant it in your memory.

Scripture Memorization Made Easy!

What is your learning style? Do you learn by hearing, by sight, or by doing?

If you learn by hearing—if you are an auditory learner—singing the Scripture memory verses, reading them aloud, or recording them and listening to your recording will be very helpful in the memorization process.

If you are a visual learner, writing the verses and repeatedly reading through them will cement them in your mind.

If you learn by doing—if you are a tactile learner—creating motions for the words or using sign language will enable you to more easily recall the verse.

After determining your learning style, link your Scripture memory with a daily task, such as driving to work, walking on a treadmill, or eating lunch. Use these daily tasks as opportunities to memorize and review your verses.

Meals at home or out with friends can be used as a time to share the verse you are memorizing with those at your table. You could close your personal email messages by typing in your weekly memory verse. Or why not say your memory verse every time you brush your teeth or put on your shoes?

The purpose of Scripture memorization is to be able to apply God's words to your life. If you memorize Scripture using methods that connect with your particular learning style, you will find it easier to hide God's Word in your heart.

—— ESTABLISHING A QUIET TIME

Like all other components of the First Place for Health program, developing a live relationship with God is not a random act. You must intentionally seek God if you are to find Him! It's not that God plays hide-and-seek with you. He is always available to you. He invites you to come boldly into His presence. He reveals Himself to you in the pages of the Bible. And once you decide to earnestly seek Him, you are sure to find Him! When you delight in Him, your gracious God will give you the desires of your heart. Spending time getting to know God involves four basic elements: a priority, a plan, a place, and practice.

A Priority

You can successfully establish a quiet time with God by making this meeting a daily priority. This may require carving out time in your day so you have time and space for this new relationship you are cultivating. Often this will mean eliminating less important things so you will have time and space to meet with God. When speaking about Jesus, John the Baptist said, "He must become greater; I must become less" (John 3:30). You will undoubtedly find that to be true as well. What might you need to eliminate from your current schedule so that spending quality time with God can become a priority?

A Plan

Having made quiet time a priority, you will want to come up with a plan. This plan will include the time you have set aside to spend with God and a general outline of how you will spend your time in God's presence.

Elements you should consider incorporating into your quiet time include:

- Singing a song of praise
- Reading a daily selection in a devotional book or reading a psalm
- Using a systematic Scripture reading plan so you will be exposed to the whole truth of God's Word
- Completing your First Place for Health Bible study for that day
- Praying—silent, spoken, and written prayer
- Writing in your spiritual journal.

You will also want to make a list of the materials you will need to make your encounter with God more meaningful:

- A Bible
- Your First Place for Health Bible study
- Your prayer journal
- A pen and/or pencil
- A devotional book
- A Bible concordance
- A college-level dictionary
- A box of tissues (tears—both of sadness and joy—are often part of our quiet time with God!)

Think of how you would plan an important business meeting or social event, and then transfer that knowledge to your meeting time with God.

A Place

Having formulated a meeting-with-God plan, you will next need to create a meeting-with-God place. Of course, God is always with you; however, in order to have quality devotional time with Him, it is desirable that you find a comfortable meeting place. You will want to select a spot that is quiet and as distraction-free as possible. Meeting with God in the same place on a regular basis will help you remember what you are there for: to have an encounter with the true and living God!

Having selected the place, put the materials you have determined to use in your quiet time into a basket or on a nearby table or shelf. Now take the time to establish your personal quiet time with God. Tailor your quiet time to fit your needs—and the time you have allotted to spend with God. Although many people elect to meet with God early in the morning, for others afternoon or evening is best. There is no hard-and-fast rule about when your quiet time should be—the only essential thing is that you establish a quiet time!

Start with a small amount of time that you know you can devote yourself to daily. You can be confident that as you consistently spend time with God each day, the amount of time you can spend will increase as you are ready for the next level of your walk with God.

I will meet with God from _____ to _____ daily.

I plan to use that time with God to _____

_____

Supplies I will need to assemble include _____

_____

My meeting place with God will be _____

_____

Practice

After you have chosen the time and place to meet God each day and you have assembled your supplies, there are four easy steps for having a fruitful and worshipful time with the Lord.

STEP 1: Clear Your Heart and Mind

"Be still, and know that I am God" (Psalm 46:10). Begin your quiet time by reading the daily Bible selection from a devotional guide or a psalm. If you are new in your Christian walk, an excellent devotional guide to use is *Streams in the Desert* by L.B. Cowman. More mature Christians might benefit from *My Utmost for His Highest* by Oswald Chambers. Of course, you can use any devotional that has a strong emphasis on Scripture and prayer.

STEP 2: Read and Interact with Scripture

"I have hidden your word in my heart that I might not sin against you" (Psalm 119:11). As you open your Bible, ask the Holy Spirit to reveal something He knows you need for this day through the reading of His Word. Always try to find a nugget to encourage or direct you through the day. As you read the passage, pay special attention to the words and phrases the Holy Spirit brings to your attention. Some words may seem to resonate in your soul. You will want to spend time meditating on the passage, asking God what lesson He is teaching you.

After reading the Scripture passage over several times, ask yourself the following questions:

- In light of what I have read today, is there something I must now do? (Confess a sin? Claim a promise? Follow an example? Obey a command? Avoid a situation?)
- How should I respond to what I've read today?

STEP 3: Pray

"Be clear minded and self-controlled so that you can pray" (1 Peter 4:7). Spend time conversing with the Lord in prayer. Prayer is such an important part of First Place for Health that there is an entire section in this member's guide devoted to the practice of prayer.

STEP 4: Praise

"Praise the LORD, O my soul, and forget not all his benefits" (Psalm 103:2). End your quiet time with a time of praise. Be sure to thank the Lord of heaven and warmth for choosing to spend time with you!

—— SHARING YOUR FAITH

Nothing is more effective in drawing someone to Jesus than sharing personal life experiences. People are more open to the good news of Jesus Christ when they see faith in action. Personal faith stories are simple and effective ways to share what Christ is doing in your life, because they show firsthand how Christ makes a difference.

Sharing your faith story has an added benefit: it builds you up in your faith, too! Is your experience in First Place for Health providing you opportunities to share with others what God is doing in your life? If you answered yes, then you have a personal faith story!

If you do not have a personal faith story, perhaps it is because you don't know Jesus Christ as your personal Lord and Savior. Read through "Steps to Becoming a Christian" (which is the next chapter) and begin today to give Christ first place in your life.

Creativity and preparation in using opportunities to share a word or story about Jesus is an important part of the Christian life. Is Jesus helping you in a special way? Are you achieving a level of success or peace that you haven't experienced in other attempts to lose weight, exercise regularly, or eat healthier? As people see you making changes and achieving success, they may ask you how you are doing it. How will—or do—you respond? Remember, your story is unique, and it may allow others to see what Christ is doing in your life. It may also help to bring Christ into the life of another person.

Personal Statements of Faith

First Place for Health gives you a great opportunity to communicate your faith and express what God is doing in your life. Be ready to use your own personal statement of faith whenever the opportunity presents itself. Personal statements of faith should be short and fit naturally into a conversation. They don't require or expect any action or response from the listener. The goal is not to get another person to change but simply to help you communicate who you are and what's important to you.

Here are some examples of short statements of faith that you might use when someone asks what you are doing to lose weight:

- "I've been meeting with a group at my church. We pray together, support each other, learn about nutrition, and study the Bible."
- "It's amazing how Bible study and prayer are helping me lose weight and eat healthier."
- "I've had a lot of support from a group I meet with at church."
- "I'm relying more on God to help me make changes in my lifestyle."

Begin keeping a list of your meaningful experiences as you go through the First Place for Health program. Also notice what is happening in the lives of others. Use the following questions to help you prepare short personal statements and stories of faith:

- What is God doing in your life physically, mentally, emotionally, and spiritually?
- How has your relationship with God changed? Is it more intimate or personal?
- How is prayer, Bible study, and/or the support of others helping you achieve your goals for a healthy weight and good nutrition?

Writing Your Personal Faith Story

Write a brief story about how God is working in your life through First Place for Health. Use your story to help you share with others what's happening in your life.

Use the following questions to help develop your story:

- Why did you join First Place for Health? What specific circumstances led you to a Christ-centered health and weight-loss program? What were you feeling when you joined?
- What was your relationship with Christ when you started First Place for Health? What is it now?
- Has your experience in First Place for Health changed your relationship with Christ? With yourself? With others?
- How has your relationship with Christ, prayer, Bible study, and group support made a difference in your life?
- What specific verse or passage of Scripture has made a difference in the way you view yourself or your relationship with Christ?
- What experiences have impacted your life since starting First Place for Health?
- In what ways is Christ working in your life today? In what ways is He meeting your needs?
- How has Christ worked in other members of your First Place for Health group?

Answer the above questions in a few sentences, and then use your answers to help you write your own short personal faith story.

MEMBER SURVEY

We would love to know more about you. Share this form with your leader.

Name _____   Birth date _____

Tell us about your family.

_____
_____
_____
_____

Would you like to receive more information   Yes   No
about our church?

What area of expertise would you be willing to share with our class?

_____
_____

Why did you join First Place for Health?

_____
_____

With notice, would you be willing to lead a Bible study   Yes   No
discussion one week?

Are you comfortable praying out loud?   _____

Would you be willing to assist recording weights and/or   Yes   No
evaluating the Live It Trackers?

Any other comments:

_____
_____

PERSONAL WEIGHT AND MEASUREMENT RECORD

WEEK	WEIGHT	+ OR -	GOAL THIS SESSION	POUNDS TO GOAL
1				
2				
3				
4				
5				
6				
7				
8				
9				
10				
11				
12				

BEGINNING MEASUREMENTS

WAIST _____ HIPS _____ THIGHS _____ CHEST _____

ENDING MEASUREMENTS

WAIST _____ HIPS _____ THIGHS _____ CHEST _____

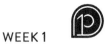
God testified concerning him: "I have found David son of Jesse, a man after my own heart; he will do everything I want him to do." Acts 13:22

Date: _____

Name: _____

Home Phone: _____

Cell Phone: _____

Email: _____

Personal Prayer Concerns

_____

_____

_____

_____

_____

_____

_____

This form is for prayer requests that are personal to you and your journey in First Place for Health. Please complete and have it ready to turn in when you arrive at your group meeting.

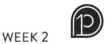
David said to the Philistine, "You come against me with sword and spear and javelin, but I come against you in the name of the LORD Almighty, the God of the armies of Israel, whom you have defied." 1 Samuel 17:45

Date: _____

Name: _____

Home Phone: _____

Cell Phone: _____

Email: _____

Personal Prayer Concerns

_____

_____

_____

_____

_____

_____

_____

This form is for prayer requests that are personal to you and your journey in First Place for Health. Please complete and have it ready to turn in when you arrive at your group meeting.

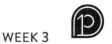

*Come, let us sing to the Lord! Let us shout joyfully to the Rock of our salvation. Let us
come to him with thanksgiving. Let us sing psalms of praise to him.*
Psalm 95:1-2 (NLT)

Date: _____

Name: _____

Home Phone: _____

Cell Phone: _____

Email: _____

Personal Prayer Concerns

_____

_____

_____

_____

_____

_____

_____

This form is for prayer requests that are personal to you and your journey in First Place for Health.
Please complete and have it ready to turn in when you arrive at your group meeting.

Sing to the Lord a new song; sing to the Lord, all the earth. Sing to the Lord, praise his name; proclaim his salvation day after day. Declare his glory among the nations, his marvelous deeds among all peoples. Psalm 96:1-3

Date: _____

Name: _____

Home Phone: _____

Cell Phone: _____

Email: _____

Personal Prayer Concerns

_____

_____

_____

_____

_____

_____

_____

This form is for prayer requests that are personal to you and your journey in First Place for Health. Please complete and have it ready to turn in when you arrive at your group meeting.

Who may ascend the mountain of the LORD? Who may stand in his holy place?
The one who has clean hands and a pure heart, who does not trust in an idol or
swear by a false god. Psalm 24:3-4

Date: _____

Name: _____

Home Phone: _____

Cell Phone: _____

Email: _____

Personal Prayer Concerns

_____

_____

_____

_____

_____

_____

_____

This form is for prayer requests that are personal to you and your journey in First Place for Health.
Please complete and have it ready to turn in when you arrive at your group meeting.

Create in me a pure heart, O God, and renew a steadfast spirit within me.
Psalm 51:10

Date: _____

Name: _____

Home Phone: _____

Cell Phone: _____

Email: _____

Personal Prayer Concerns

_____

_____

_____

_____

_____

_____

_____

_____

This form is for prayer requests that are personal to you and your journey in First Place for Health. Please complete and have it ready to turn in when you arrive at your group meeting.

For he knows how we are formed, he remembers that we are dust.
Psalm 103:14

Date: _____

Name: _____

Home Phone: _____

Cell Phone: _____

Email: _____

Personal Prayer Concerns

_____

_____

_____

_____

_____

_____

_____

This form is for prayer requests that are personal to you and your journey in First Place for Health.
Please complete and have it ready to turn in when you arrive at your group meeting.

I am the Root and the Offspring of David, and the bright Morning Star.
Revelation 22:16

Date: _____

Name: _____

Home Phone: _____

Cell Phone: _____

Email: _____

Personal Prayer Concern

_____

_____

_____

_____

_____

_____

_____

This form is for prayer requests that are personal to you and your journey in First Place for Health. Please complete and have it ready to turn in when you arrive at your group meeting.

Date: _____

Name: _____

Home Phone: _____

Cell Phone: _____

Email: _____

Personal Prayer Concerns

_____

_____

_____

_____

_____

_____

_____

_____

This form is for prayer requests that are personal to you and your journey in First Place for Health. Please complete and have it ready to turn in when you arrive at your group meeting.

LIVE IT TRACKER

Name: _____   Date: _____ Week #: _____

My activity goal for next week: loss/gain _____ Calorie Range: _____
○ None   ○ <30 min/day   ○ 30-60 min/day
                                               My week at a glance:
                                               ○ Great   ○ So-so   ○ Not so great
My food goal for next week: _____
_____   Activity level:
                                               ○ None   ○ <30 min/day   ○ 30-60 min/day

RECOMMENDED DAILY AMOUNT OF FOOD FROM EACH GROUP

GROUP	DAILY CALORIES							
	1300-1400	1500-1600	1700-1800	1900-2000	2100-2200	2300-2400	2500-2600	2700-2800
Fruits	1.5 – 2 c.	1.5 – 2 c.	1.5 – 2 c.	2 – 2.5 c.	2 – 2.5 c.	2.5 – 3.5 c.	3.5 – 4.5 c.	3.5 – 4.5 c.
Vegetables	1.5 – 2 c.	2 – 2.5 c.	2.5 – 3 c.	2.5 – 3 c.	3 – 3.5 c.	3.5 – 4.5 c.	4.5 – 5 c.	4.5 – 5 c.
Grains	5 oz eq.	5-6 oz eq.	6-7 oz eq.	6-7 oz eq.	7-8 oz eq.	8-9 oz eq.	9-10 oz eq.	10-11 oz eq.
Dairy	2-3 c.	3 c.	3 c.	3 c.	3 c.	3 c.	3 c.	3 c.
Protein	4 oz eq.	5 oz eq.	5-5.5 oz eq.	5.5-6.5 oz eq.	6.5-7 oz eq.	7-7.5 oz eq.	7-7.5 oz eq.	7.5-8 oz eq.
Healthy Oils & Other Fats	4 tsp.	5 tsp.	5 tsp.	6 tsp.	6 tsp.	7 tsp.	8 tsp.	8 tsp.
Water & Super Beverages*	Women: 9 c. Men: 13 c.	Women: 9 c. Men: 13 c.	Women: 9 c. Men: 13 c.	Women: 9 c. Men: 13 c.	Women: 9 c. Men: 13 c.	Women: 9 c. Men: 13 c.	Women: 9 c. Men: 13 c.	Women: 9 c. Men: 13 c.

*May count up to 3 cups caffeinated tea or coffee toward goal

DAILY FOOD GROUP TRACKER

	GROUP	FRUITS	VEGETABLES	GRAINS	PROTEIN	DAIRY	HEALTHY OILS & OTHER FATS	WATER & SUPER BEVERAGES
1	Estimate Total							
2	Estimate Total							
3	Estimate Total							
4	Estimate Total							
5	Estimate Total							
6	Estimate Total							
7	Estimate Total							

FOOD CHOICES   DAY ❶

Breakfast: _____
Lunch: _____
Dinner: _____
Snacks: _____

PHYSICAL ACTIVITY   steps/miles/minutes: _____   ### SPIRITUAL ACTIVITY
description: _____   description: _____

FOOD CHOICES

DAY ❷

Breakfast: _____
Lunch: _____
Dinner: _____
Snacks: _____

PHYSICAL ACTIVITY   steps/miles/minutes: _____

description: _____

SPIRITUAL ACTIVITY

description: _____

FOOD CHOICES

DAY ❸

Breakfast: _____
Lunch: _____
Dinner: _____
Snacks: _____

PHYSICAL ACTIVITY   steps/miles/minutes: _____

description: _____

SPIRITUAL ACTIVITY

description: _____

FOOD CHOICES

DAY ❹

Breakfast: _____
Lunch: _____
Dinner: _____
Snacks: _____

PHYSICAL ACTIVITY   steps/miles/minutes: _____

description: _____

SPIRITUAL ACTIVITY

description: _____

FOOD CHOICES

DAY ❺

Breakfast: _____
Lunch: _____
Dinner: _____
Snacks: _____

PHYSICAL ACTIVITY   steps/miles/minutes: _____

description: _____

SPIRITUAL ACTIVITY

description: _____

FOOD CHOICES

DAY ❻

Breakfast: _____
Lunch: _____
Dinner: _____
Snacks: _____

PHYSICAL ACTIVITY   steps/miles/minutes: _____

description: _____

SPIRITUAL ACTIVITY

description: _____

FOOD CHOICES

DAY ❼

Breakfast: _____
Lunch: _____
Dinner: _____
Snacks: _____

PHYSICAL ACTIVITY   steps/miles/minutes: _____

description: _____

SPIRITUAL ACTIVITY

description: _____

LIVE IT TRACKER

Name: _____

Date: _____ Week #: _____

My activity goal for next week:
- ○ None   ○ <30 min/day   ○ 30-60 min/day

loss / gain _____ Calorie Range: _____

My week at a glance:
- ○ Great   ○ So-so   ○ Not so great

My food goal for next week: _____
_____

Activity level:
- ○ None   ○ <30 min/day   ○ 30-60 min/day

RECOMMENDED DAILY AMOUNT OF FOOD FROM EACH GROUP

GROUP	DAILY CALORIES							
	1300-1400	1500-1600	1700-1800	1900-2000	2100-2200	2300-2400	2500-2600	2700-2800
Fruits	1.5 – 2 c.	1.5 – 2 c.	1.5 – 2 c.	2 – 2.5 c.	2 – 2.5 c.	2.5 – 3.5 c.	3.5 – 4.5 c.	3.5 – 4.5 c.
Vegetables	1.5 – 2 c.	2 – 2.5 c.	2.5 – 3 c.	2.5 – 3 c.	3 – 3.5 c.	3.5 – 4.5 c..	4.5 – 5 c.	4.5 – 5 c.
Grains	5 oz eq.	5-6 oz eq.	6-7 oz eq.	6-7 oz eq.	7-8 oz eq.	8-9 oz eq.	9-10 oz eq.	10-11 oz eq.
Dairy	2-3 c.	3 c.	3 c.	3 c.	3 c.	3 c.	3 c.	3 c.
Protein	4 oz eq.	5 oz eq.	5-5.5 oz eq.	5.5-6.5 oz eq.	6.5-7 oz eq.	7-7.5 oz eq.	7-7.5 oz eq.	7.5-8 oz eq.
Healthy Oils & Other Fats	4 tsp.	5 tsp.	5 tsp.	6 tsp.	6 tsp.	7 tsp.	8 tsp.	8 tsp.
Water & Super Beverages*	Women: 9 c. Men: 13 c.	Women: 9 c. Men: 13 c.	Women: 9 c. Men: 13 c.	Women: 9 c. Men: 13 c.	Women: 9 c. Men: 13 c.	Women: 9 c. Men: 13 c.	Women: 9 c. Men: 13 c.	Women: 9 c. Men: 13 c.

*May count up to 3 cups caffeinated tea or coffee toward goal

DAILY FOOD GROUP TRACKER

GROUP	FRUITS	VEGETABLES	GRAINS	PROTEIN	DAIRY	HEALTHY OILS & OTHER FATS	WATER & SUPER BEVERAGES
❶ Estimate Total							
❷ Estimate Total							
❸ Estimate Total							
❹ Estimate Total							
❺ Estimate Total							
❻ Estimate Total							
❼ Estimate Total							

FOOD CHOICES   DAY ❶

Breakfast: _____
Lunch: _____
Dinner: _____
Snacks: _____

PHYSICAL ACTIVITY steps/miles/minutes: _____

SPIRITUAL ACTIVITY

description: _____

description: _____

FOOD CHOICES DAY ❷

Breakfast: _____
Lunch: _____
Dinner: _____
Snacks: _____

PHYSICAL ACTIVITY   steps/miles/minutes: _____

description: _____

SPIRITUAL ACTIVITY

description: _____

FOOD CHOICES DAY ❸

Breakfast: _____
Lunch: _____
Dinner: _____
Snacks: _____

PHYSICAL ACTIVITY   steps/miles/minutes: _____

description: _____

SPIRITUAL ACTIVITY

description: _____

FOOD CHOICES DAY ❹

Breakfast: _____
Lunch: _____
Dinner: _____
Snacks: _____

PHYSICAL ACTIVITY   steps/miles/minutes: _____

description: _____

SPIRITUAL ACTIVITY

description: _____

FOOD CHOICES DAY ❺

Breakfast: _____
Lunch: _____
Dinner: _____
Snacks: _____

PHYSICAL ACTIVITY   steps/miles/minutes: _____

description: _____

SPIRITUAL ACTIVITY

description: _____

FOOD CHOICES DAY ❻

Breakfast: _____
Lunch: _____
Dinner: _____
Snacks: _____

PHYSICAL ACTIVITY   steps/miles/minutes: _____

description: _____

SPIRITUAL ACTIVITY

description: _____

FOOD CHOICES DAY ❼

Breakfast: _____
Lunch: _____
Dinner: _____
Snacks: _____

PHYSICAL ACTIVITY   steps/miles/minutes: _____

description: _____

SPIRITUAL ACTIVITY

description: _____

LIVE IT TRACKER

Name: _____

Date: _____ Week #: _____

My activity goal for next week:
○ None   ○ <30 min/day   ○ 30-60 min/day

loss/gain _____ Calorie Range: _____

My week at a glance:
○ Great   ○ So-so   ○ Not so great

My food goal for next week: _____

Activity level:
○ None   ○ <30 min/day   ○ 30-60 min/day

RECOMMENDED DAILY AMOUNT OF FOOD FROM EACH GROUP

GROUP	DAILY CALORIES							
	1300-1400	1500-1600	1700-1800	1900-2000	2100-2200	2300-2400	2500-2600	2700-2800
Fruits	1.5 – 2 c.	1.5 – 2 c.	1.5 – 2 c.	2 – 2.5 c.	2 – 2.5 c.	2.5 – 3.5 c.	3.5 – 4.5 c.	3.5 – 4.5 c.
Vegetables	1.5 – 2 c.	2 – 2.5 c.	2.5 – 3 c.	2.5 – 3 c.	3 – 3.5 c.	3.5 – 4.5 c.	4.5 – 5 c.	4.5 – 5 c.
Grains	5 oz eq.	5-6 oz eq.	6-7 oz eq.	6-7 oz eq.	7-8 oz eq.	8-9 oz eq.	9-10 oz eq.	10-11 oz eq.
Dairy	2-3 c.	3 c.	3 c.	3 c.	3 c.	3 c.	3 c.	3 c.
Protein	4 oz eq.	5 oz eq.	5-5.5 oz eq.	5.5-6.5 oz eq.	6.5-7 oz eq.	7-7.5 oz eq.	7-7.5 oz eq.	7.5-8 oz eq.
Healthy Oils & Other Fats	4 tsp.	5 tsp.	5 tsp.	6 tsp.	6 tsp.	7 tsp.	8 tsp.	8 tsp.
Water & Super Beverages*	Women: 9 c. Men: 13 c.	Women: 9 c. Men: 13 c.	Women: 9 c. Men: 13 c.	Women: 9 c. Men: 13 c.	Women: 9 c. Men: 13 c.	Women: 9 c. Men: 13 c.	Women: 9 c. Men: 13 c.	Women: 9 c. Men: 13 c.

*May count up to 3 cups caffeinated tea or coffee toward goal

DAILY FOOD GROUP TRACKER

GROUP	FRUITS	VEGETABLES	GRAINS	PROTEIN	DAIRY	HEALTHY OILS & OTHER FATS	WATER & SUPER BEVERAGES
① Estimate Total							
② Estimate Total							
③ Estimate Total							
④ Estimate Total							
⑤ Estimate Total							
⑥ Estimate Total							
⑦ Estimate Total							

FOOD CHOICES   DAY ①

Breakfast: _____
Lunch: _____
Dinner: _____
Snacks: _____

PHYSICAL ACTIVITY   steps/miles/minutes: _____

description: _____

SPIRITUAL ACTIVITY

description: _____

FOOD CHOICES DAY ❷

Breakfast: _____
Lunch: _____
Dinner: _____
Snacks: _____

PHYSICAL ACTIVITY steps/miles/minutes: _____

description: _____

SPIRITUAL ACTIVITY

description: _____

FOOD CHOICES DAY ❸

Breakfast: _____
Lunch: _____
Dinner: _____
Snacks: _____

PHYSICAL ACTIVITY steps/miles/minutes: _____

description: _____

SPIRITUAL ACTIVITY

description: _____

FOOD CHOICES DAY ❹

Breakfast: _____
Lunch: _____
Dinner: _____
Snacks: _____

PHYSICAL ACTIVITY steps/miles/minutes: _____

description: _____

SPIRITUAL ACTIVITY

description: _____

FOOD CHOICES DAY ❺

Breakfast: _____
Lunch: _____
Dinner: _____
Snacks: _____

PHYSICAL ACTIVITY steps/miles/minutes: _____

description: _____

SPIRITUAL ACTIVITY

description: _____

FOOD CHOICES DAY ❻

Breakfast: _____
Lunch: _____
Dinner: _____
Snacks: _____

PHYSICAL ACTIVITY steps/miles/minutes: _____

description: _____

SPIRITUAL ACTIVITY

description: _____

FOOD CHOICES DAY ❼

Breakfast: _____
Lunch: _____
Dinner: _____
Snacks: _____

PHYSICAL ACTIVITY steps/miles/minutes: _____

description: _____

SPIRITUAL ACTIVITY

description: _____

LIVE IT TRACKER

Name: _____

Date: _____ Week #: _____

My activity goal for next week:
○ None ○ <30 min/day ○ 30-60 min/day

loss/gain _____ Calorie Range: _____

My food goal for next week: _____

My week at a glance:
○ Great ○ So-so ○ Not so great

Activity level:
○ None ○ <30 min/day ○ 30-60 min/day

RECOMMENDED DAILY AMOUNT OF FOOD FROM EACH GROUP

GROUP	DAILY CALORIES							
	1300-1400	1500-1600	1700-1800	1900-2000	2100-2200	2300-2400	2500-2600	2700-2800
Fruits	1.5 – 2 c.	1.5 – 2 c.	1.5 – 2 c.	2 – 2.5 c.	2 – 2.5 c.	2.5 – 3.5 c.	3.5 – 4.5 c.	3.5 – 4.5 c.
Vegetables	1.5 – 2 c.	2 – 2.5 c.	2.5 – 3 c.	2.5 – 3 c.	3 – 3.5 c.	3.5 – 4.5 c.	4.5 – 5 c.	4.5 – 5 c.
Grains	5 oz eq.	5-6 oz eq.	6-7 oz eq.	6-7 oz eq.	7-8 oz eq.	8-9 oz eq.	9-10 oz eq.	10-11 oz eq.
Dairy	2-3 c.	3 c.	3 c.	3 c.	3 c.	3 c.	3 c.	3 c.
Protein	4 oz eq.	5 oz eq.	5-5.5 oz eq.	5.5-6.5 oz eq.	6.5-7 oz eq.	7-7.5 oz eq.	7-7.5 oz eq.	7.5-8 oz eq.
Healthy Oils & Other Fats	4 tsp.	5 tsp.	5 tsp.	6 tsp.	6 tsp.	7 tsp.	8 tsp.	8 tsp.
Water & Super Beverages*	Women: 9 c. Men: 13 c.	Women: 9 c. Men: 13 c.	Women: 9 c. Men: 13 c.	Women: 9 c. Men: 13 c.	Women: 9 c. Men: 13 c.	Women: 9 c. Men: 13 c.	Women: 9 c. Men: 13 c.	Women: 9 c. Men: 13 c.

*May count up to 3 cups caffeinated tea or coffee toward goal

DAILY FOOD GROUP TRACKER

GROUP	FRUITS	VEGETABLES	GRAINS	PROTEIN	DAIRY	HEALTHY OILS & OTHER FATS	WATER & SUPER BEVERAGES
1 Estimate Total							
2 Estimate Total							
3 Estimate Total							
4 Estimate Total							
5 Estimate Total							
6 Estimate Total							
7 Estimate Total							

FOOD CHOICES

Breakfast: _____
Lunch: _____
Dinner: _____
Snacks: _____

DAY ❶

PHYSICAL ACTIVITY steps/miles/minutes: _____
description: _____

SPIRITUAL ACTIVITY
description: _____

FOOD CHOICES   DAY 2

Breakfast: _____
Lunch: _____
Dinner: _____
Snacks: _____

PHYSICAL ACTIVITY   steps/miles/minutes: _____   SPIRITUAL ACTIVITY

description: _____   description: _____

FOOD CHOICES   DAY 3

Breakfast: _____
Lunch: _____
Dinner: _____
Snacks: _____

PHYSICAL ACTIVITY   steps/miles/minutes: _____   SPIRITUAL ACTIVITY

description: _____   description: _____

FOOD CHOICES   DAY 4

Breakfast: _____
Lunch: _____
Dinner: _____
Snacks: _____

PHYSICAL ACTIVITY   steps/miles/minutes: _____   SPIRITUAL ACTIVITY

description: _____   description: _____

FOOD CHOICES   DAY 5

Breakfast: _____
Lunch: _____
Dinner: _____
Snacks: _____

PHYSICAL ACTIVITY   steps/miles/minutes: _____   SPIRITUAL ACTIVITY

description: _____   description: _____

FOOD CHOICES   DAY 6

Breakfast: _____
Lunch: _____
Dinner: _____
Snacks: _____

PHYSICAL ACTIVITY   steps/miles/minutes: _____   SPIRITUAL ACTIVITY

description: _____   description: _____

FOOD CHOICES   DAY 7

Breakfast: _____
Lunch: _____
Dinner: _____
Snacks: _____

PHYSICAL ACTIVITY   steps/miles/minutes: _____   SPIRITUAL ACTIVITY

description: _____   description: _____

LIVE IT TRACKER

Name: _____

Date: _____ Week #: _____

My activity goal for next week:
○ None   ○ <30 min/day   ○ 30-60 min/day

loss/gain _____ Calorie Range: _____

My week at a glance:
○ Great   ○ So-so   ○ Not so great

My food goal for next week: _____

Activity level:
○ None   ○ <30 min/day   ○ 30-60 min/day

RECOMMENDED DAILY AMOUNT OF FOOD FROM EACH GROUP

GROUP	DAILY CALORIES							
	1300-1400	1500-1600	1700-1800	1900-2000	2100-2200	2300-2400	2500-2600	2700-2800
Fruits	1.5 - 2 c.	1.5 - 2 c.	1.5 - 2 c.	2 - 2.5 c.	2 - 2.5 c.	2.5 - 3.5 c.	3.5 - 4.5 c.	3.5 - 4.5 c.
Vegetables	1.5 - 2 c.	2 - 2.5 c.	2.5 - 3 c.	2.5 - 3 c.	3 - 3.5 c.	3.5 - 4.5 c.	4.5 - 5 c.	4.5 - 5 c.
Grains	5 oz eq.	5-6 oz eq.	6-7 oz eq.	6-7 oz eq.	7-8 oz eq.	8-9 oz eq.	9-10 oz eq.	10-11 oz eq.
Dairy	2-3 c.	3 c.	3 c.	3 c.	3 c.	3 c.	3 c.	3 c.
Protein	4 oz eq.	5 oz eq	5-5.5 oz eq.	5.5-6.5 oz eq.	6.5-7 oz eq.	7-7.5 oz eq.	7-7.5 oz eq.	7.5-8 oz eq.
Healthy Oils & Other Fats	4 tsp.	5 tsp.	5 tsp.	6 tsp.	6 tsp.	7 tsp.	8 tsp.	8 tsp.
Water & Super Beverages*	Women: 9 c. Men: 13 c.	Women: 9 c. Men: 13 c.	Women: 9 c. Men: 13 c.	Women: 9 c. Men: 13 c.	Women: 9 c. Men: 13 c.	Women: 9 c. Men: 13 c.	Women: 9 c. Men: 13 c.	Women: 9 c. Men: 13 c.

*May count up to 3 cups caffeinated tea or coffee toward goal

DAILY FOOD GROUP TRACKER

GROUP	FRUITS	VEGETABLES	GRAINS	PROTEIN	DAIRY	HEALTHY OILS & OTHER FATS	WATER & SUPER BEVERAGES
1 Estimate Total							
2 Estimate Total							
3 Estimate Total							
4 Estimate Total							
5 Estimate Total							
6 Estimate Total							
7 Estimate Total							

FOOD CHOICES   DAY ❶

Breakfast: _____
Lunch: _____
Dinner: _____
Snacks: _____

PHYSICAL ACTIVITY   steps/miles/minutes: _____

SPIRITUAL ACTIVITY

description: _____

description: _____

FOOD CHOICES   DAY ❷

Breakfast: _____

Lunch: _____

Dinner: _____

Snacks: _____

PHYSICAL ACTIVITY   steps/miles/minutes: _____   ### SPIRITUAL ACTIVITY

description: _____   description: _____

FOOD CHOICES   DAY ❸

Breakfast: _____

Lunch: _____

Dinner: _____

Snacks: _____

PHYSICAL ACTIVITY   steps/miles/minutes: _____   ### SPIRITUAL ACTIVITY

description: _____   description: _____

FOOD CHOICES   DAY ❹

Breakfast: _____

Lunch: _____

Dinner: _____

Snacks: _____

PHYSICAL ACTIVITY   steps/miles/minutes: _____   ### SPIRITUAL ACTIVITY

description: _____   description: _____

FOOD CHOICES   DAY ❺

Breakfast: _____

Lunch: _____

Dinner: _____

Snacks: _____

PHYSICAL ACTIVITY   steps/miles/minutes: _____   ### SPIRITUAL ACTIVITY

description: _____   description: _____

FOOD CHOICES   DAY ❻

Breakfast: _____

Lunch: _____

Dinner: _____

Snacks: _____

PHYSICAL ACTIVITY   steps/miles/minutes: _____   ### SPIRITUAL ACTIVITY

description: _____   description: _____

FOOD CHOICES   DAY ❼

Breakfast: _____

Lunch: _____

Dinner: _____

Snacks: _____

PHYSICAL ACTIVITY   steps/miles/minutes: _____   ### SPIRITUAL ACTIVITY

description: _____   description: _____

LIVE IT TRACKER

RECOMMENDED DAILY AMOUNT OF FOOD FROM EACH GROUP

GROUP	DAILY CALORIES							
	1300-1400	1500-1600	1700-1800	1900-2000	2100-2200	2300-2400	2500-2600	2700-2800
Fruits	1.5 – 2 c.	1.5 – 2 c.	1.5 – 2 c.	2 – 2.5 c.	2 – 2.5 c.	2.5 – 3.5 c.	3.5 – 4.5 c.	3.5 – 4.5 c.
Vegetables	1.5 – 2 c.	2 – 2.5 c.	2.5 – 3 c.	2.5 – 3 c.	3 – 3.5 c.	3.5 – 4.5 c..	4.5 – 5 c.	4.5 – 5 c.
Grains	5 oz eq.	5-6 oz eq.	6-7 oz eq.	6-7 oz eq.	7-8 oz eq.	8-9 oz eq.	9-10 oz eq.	10-11 oz eq.
Dairy	2-3 c.	3 c.	3 c.	3 c.	3 c.	3 c.	3 c.	3 c.
Protein	4 oz eq.	5 oz eq.	5-5.5 oz eq.	5.5-6.5 oz eq.	6.5-7 oz eq.	7-7.5 oz eq.	7-7.5 oz eq.	7.5-8 oz eq.
Healthy Oils & Other Fats	4 tsp.	5 tsp.	5 tsp.	6 tsp.	6 tsp.	7 tsp.	8 tsp.	8 tsp.
Water & Super Beverages*	Women: 9 c. Men: 13 c.	Women: 9 c. Men: 13 c.	Women: 9 c. Men: 13 c.	Women: 9 c. Men: 13 c.	Women: 9 c. Men: 13 c.	Women: 9 c. Men: 13 c.	Women: 9 c. Men: 13 c.	Women: 9 c. Men: 13 c.

*May count up to 3 cups caffeinated tea or coffee toward goal

DAILY FOOD GROUP TRACKER

GROUP	FRUITS	VEGETABLES	GRAINS	PROTEIN	DAIRY	HEALTHY OILS & OTHER FATS	WATER & SUPER BEVERAGES
1 Estimate Total							
2 Estimate Total							
3 Estimate Total							
4 Estimate Total							
5 Estimate Total							
6 Estimate Total							
7 Estimate Total							

FOOD CHOICES   DAY ❶

Breakfast: _____
Lunch: _____
Dinner: _____
Snacks: _____

PHYSICAL ACTIVITY   steps/miles/minutes: _____   **SPIRITUAL ACTIVITY**

description: _____   description: _____
_____   _____

FOOD CHOICES   DAY ❷

Breakfast: _____
Lunch: _____
Dinner: _____
Snacks: _____

PHYSICAL ACTIVITY   steps/miles/minutes: _____   ### SPIRITUAL ACTIVITY

description: _____   description: _____

FOOD CHOICES   DAY ❸

Breakfast: _____
Lunch: _____
Dinner: _____
Snacks: _____

PHYSICAL ACTIVITY   steps/miles/minutes: _____   ### SPIRITUAL ACTIVITY

description: _____   description: _____

FOOD CHOICES   DAY ❹

Breakfast: _____
Lunch: _____
Dinner: _____
Snacks: _____

PHYSICAL ACTIVITY   steps/miles/minutes: _____   ### SPIRITUAL ACTIVITY

description: _____   description: _____

FOOD CHOICES   DAY ❺

Breakfast: _____
Lunch: _____
Dinner: _____
Snacks: _____

PHYSICAL ACTIVITY   steps/miles/minutes: _____   ### SPIRITUAL ACTIVITY

description: _____   description: _____

FOOD CHOICES   DAY ❻

Breakfast: _____
Lunch: _____
Dinner: _____
Snacks: _____

PHYSICAL ACTIVITY   steps/miles/minutes: _____   ### SPIRITUAL ACTIVITY

description: _____   description: _____

FOOD CHOICES   DAY ❼

Breakfast: _____
Lunch: _____
Dinner: _____
Snacks: _____

PHYSICAL ACTIVITY   steps/miles/minutes: _____   ### SPIRITUAL ACTIVITY

description: _____   description: _____

LIVE IT TRACKER

Name: _____   Date: _____ Week #: _____

My activity goal for next week: loss / gain _____ Calorie Range: _____
○ None   ○ <30 min/day   ○ 30-60 min/day

My week at a glance:
○ Great   ○ So-so   ○ Not so great

My food goal for next week: _____

Activity level:
○ None   ○ <30 min/day   ○ 30-60 min/day

RECOMMENDED DAILY AMOUNT OF FOOD FROM EACH GROUP

GROUP	DAILY CALORIES							
	1300-1400	1500-1600	1700-1800	1900-2000	2100-2200	2300-2400	2500-2600	2700-2800
Fruits	1.5 - 2 c.	1.5 - 2 c.	1.5 - 2 c.	2 - 2.5 c.	2 - 2.5 c.	2.5 - 3.5 c.	3.5 - 4.5 c.	3.5 - 4.5 c.
Vegetables	1.5 - 2 c.	2 - 2.5 c.	2.5 - 3 c.	2.5 - 3 c.	3 - 3.5 c.	3.5 - 4.5 c.	4.5 - 5 c.	4.5 - 5 c.
Grains	5 oz eq.	5-6 oz eq.	6-7 oz eq.	6-7 oz eq.	7-8 oz eq.	8-9 oz eq.	9-10 oz eq.	10-11 oz eq.
Dairy	2-3 c.	3 c.	3 c.	3 c.	3 c.	3 c.	3 c.	3 c.
Protein	4 oz eq.	5 oz eq.	5-5.5 oz eq.	5.5-6.5 oz eq.	6.5-7 oz eq.	7-7.5 oz eq.	7-7.5 oz eq.	7.5-8 oz eq.
Healthy Oils & Other Fats	4 tsp.	5 tsp.	5 tsp.	6 tsp.	6 tsp.	7 tsp.	8 tsp.	8 tsp.
Water & Super Beverages*	Women: 9 c. Men: 13 c.	Women: 9 c. Men: 13 c.	Women: 9 c. Men: 13 c.	Women: 9 c. Men: 13 c.	Women: 9 c. Men: 13 c.	Women: 9 c. Men: 13 c.	Women: 9 c. Men: 13 c.	Women: 9 c. Men: 13 c.

*May count up to 3 cups caffeinated tea or coffee toward goal

DAILY FOOD GROUP TRACKER

GROUP	FRUITS	VEGETABLES	GRAINS	PROTEIN	DAIRY	HEALTHY OILS & OTHER FATS	WATER & SUPER BEVERAGES
1 Estimate Total							
2 Estimate Total							
3 Estimate Total							
4 Estimate Total							
5 Estimate Total							
6 Estimate Total							
7 Estimate Total							

FOOD CHOICES   DAY ❶

Breakfast: _____
Lunch: _____
Dinner: _____
Snacks: _____

PHYSICAL ACTIVITY   steps/miles/minutes: _____   **SPIRITUAL ACTIVITY**

description: _____   description: _____

FOOD CHOICES

DAY 2

Breakfast: _____
Lunch: _____
Dinner: _____
Snacks: _____

PHYSICAL ACTIVITY   steps/miles/minutes: _____

description: _____

SPIRITUAL ACTIVITY

description: _____

FOOD CHOICES

DAY 3

Breakfast: _____
Lunch: _____
Dinner: _____
Snacks: _____

PHYSICAL ACTIVITY   steps/miles/minutes: _____

description: _____

SPIRITUAL ACTIVITY

description: _____

FOOD CHOICES

DAY 4

Breakfast: _____
Lunch: _____
Dinner: _____
Snacks: _____

PHYSICAL ACTIVITY   steps/miles/minutes: _____

description: _____

SPIRITUAL ACTIVITY

description: _____

FOOD CHOICES

DAY 5

Breakfast: _____
Lunch: _____
Dinner: _____
Snacks: _____

PHYSICAL ACTIVITY   steps/miles/minutes: _____

description: _____

SPIRITUAL ACTIVITY

description: _____

FOOD CHOICES

DAY 6

Breakfast: _____
Lunch: _____
Dinner: _____
Snacks: _____

PHYSICAL ACTIVITY   steps/miles/minutes: _____

description: _____

SPIRITUAL ACTIVITY

description: _____

FOOD CHOICES

DAY 7

Breakfast: _____
Lunch: _____
Dinner: _____
Snacks: _____

PHYSICAL ACTIVITY   steps/miles/minutes: _____

description: _____

SPIRITUAL ACTIVITY

description: _____

LIVE IT TRACKER

Name: _____   Date: _____ Week #: _____

My activity goal for next week:

○ None   ○ <30 min/day   ○ 30-60 min/day

loss/gain _____   Calorie Range: _____

My week at a glance:

○ Great   ○ So-so   ○ Not so great

My food goal for next week: _____

Activity level:

○ None   ○ <30 min/day   ○ 30-60 min/day

RECOMMENDED DAILY AMOUNT OF FOOD FROM EACH GROUP

GROUP	DAILY CALORIES							
......	1300-1400	1500-1600	1700-1800	1900-2000	2100-2200	2300-2400	2500-2600	2700-2800
Fruits	1.5 – 2 c.	1.5 – 2 c.	1.5 – 2 c.	2 – 2.5 c.	2 – 2.5 c.	2.5 – 3.5 c.	3.5 – 4.5 c.	3.5 – 4.5 c.
Vegetables	1.5 – 2 c.	2 – 2.5 c.	2.5 – 3 c.	2.5 – 3 c.	3 – 3.5 c.	3.5 – 4.5 c.	4.5 – 5 c.	4.5 – 5 c.
Grains	5 oz eq.	5-6 oz eq.	6-7 oz eq.	6-7 oz eq.	7-8 oz eq.	8-9 oz eq	9-10 oz eq.	10-11 oz eq.
Dairy	2-3 c.	3 c.	3 c.	3 c.	3 c.	3 c.	3 c.	3 c.
Protein	4 oz eq.	5 oz eq.	5-5.5 oz eq.	5.5-6.5 oz eq.	6.5-7 oz eq.	7-7.5 oz eq.	7-7.5 oz eq.	7.5-8 oz eq.
Healthy Oils & Other Fats	4 tsp.	5 tsp.	5 tsp.	6 tsp.	6 tsp.	7 tsp.	8 tsp.	8 tsp.
Water & Super Beverages*	Women: 9 c. Men: 13 c.	Women: 9 c. Men: 13 c.	Women: 9 c. Men: 13 c.	Women: 9 c. Men: 13 c.	Women: 9 c. Men: 13 c.	Women: 9 c. Men: 13 c.	Women: 9 c. Men: 13 c.	Women: 9 c. Men: 13 c.

*May count up to 3 cups caffeinated tea or coffee toward goal

DAILY FOOD GROUP TRACKER

GROUP	FRUITS	VEGETABLES	GRAINS	PROTEIN	DAIRY	HEALTHY OILS & OTHER FATS	WATER & SUPER BEVERAGES
1 Estimate Total							
2 Estimate Total							
3 Estimate Total							
4 Estimate Total							
5 Estimate Total							
6 Estimate Total							
7 Estimate Total							

FOOD CHOICES   DAY ❶

Breakfast: _____

Lunch: _____

Dinner: _____

Snacks: _____

PHYSICAL ACTIVITY   steps/miles/minutes: _____   **SPIRITUAL ACTIVITY**

description: _____   description: _____

FOOD CHOICES

DAY ❷

Breakfast: _____
Lunch: _____
Dinner: _____
Snacks: _____

PHYSICAL ACTIVITY   steps/miles/minutes: _____

description: _____

SPIRITUAL ACTIVITY

description: _____

FOOD CHOICES

DAY ❸

Breakfast: _____
Lunch: _____
Dinner: _____
Snacks: _____

PHYSICAL ACTIVITY   steps/miles/minutes: _____

description: _____

SPIRITUAL ACTIVITY

description: _____

FOOD CHOICES

DAY ❹

Breakfast: _____
Lunch: _____
Dinner: _____
Snacks: _____

PHYSICAL ACTIVITY   steps/miles/minutes: _____

description: _____

SPIRITUAL ACTIVITY

description: _____

FOOD CHOICES

DAY ❺

Breakfast: _____
Lunch: _____
Dinner: _____
Snacks: _____

PHYSICAL ACTIVITY   steps/miles/minutes: _____

description: _____

SPIRITUAL ACTIVITY

description: _____

FOOD CHOICES

DAY ❻

Breakfast: _____
Lunch: _____
Dinner: _____
Snacks: _____

PHYSICAL ACTIVITY   steps/miles/minutes: _____

description: _____

SPIRITUAL ACTIVITY

description: _____

FOOD CHOICES

DAY ❼

Breakfast: _____
Lunch: _____
Dinner: _____
Snacks: _____

PHYSICAL ACTIVITY   steps/miles/minutes: _____

description: _____

SPIRITUAL ACTIVITY

description: _____

LIVE IT TRACKER

Name: _____

Date: _____ Week #: _____

My activity goal for next week:
○ None ○ <30 min/day ○ 30-60 min/day

loss / gain _____ Calorie Range: _____

My week at a glance:
○ Great ○ So-so ○ Not so great

My food goal for next week: _____
_____

Activity level:
○ None ○ <30 min/day ○ 30-60 min/day

RECOMMENDED DAILY AMOUNT OF FOOD FROM EACH GROUP

GROUP	DAILY CALORIES							
	1300-1400	1500-1600	1700-1800	1900-2000	2100-2200	2300-2400	2500-2600	2700-2800
Fruits	1.5 - 2 c.	1.5 - 2 c.	1.5 - 2 c.	2 - 2.5 c.	2 - 2.5 c.	2.5 - 3.5 c.	3.5 - 4.5 c.	3.5 - 4.5 c.
Vegetables	1.5 - 2 c.	2 - 2.5 c.	2.5 - 3 c.	2.5 - 3 c.	3 - 3.5 c.	3.5 - 4.5 c.	4.5 - 5 c.	4.5 - 5 c.
Grains	5 oz eq.	5-6 oz eq.	6-7 oz eq.	6-7 oz eq.	7-8 oz eq.	8-9 oz eq.	9-10 oz eq.	10-11 oz eq.
Dairy	2-3 c.	3 c.	3 c.	3 c.	3 c.	3 c.	3 c.	3 c.
Protein	4 oz eq.	5 oz eq.	5-5.5 oz eq.	5.5-6.5 oz eq.	6.5-7 oz eq.	7-7.5 oz eq.	7-7.5 oz eq.	7.5-8 oz eq.
Healthy Oils & Other Fats	4 tsp.	5 tsp.	5 tsp.	6 tsp.	6 tsp.	7 tsp.	8 tsp.	8 tsp.
Water & Super Beverages*	Women: 9 c. Men: 13 c.	Women: 9 c. Men: 13 c.	Women: 9 c. Men: 13 c.	Women: 9 c. Men: 13 c.	Women: 9 c. Men: 13 c.	Women: 9 c. Men: 13 c.	Women: 9 c. Men: 13 c.	Women: 9 c. Men: 13 c.

*May count up to 3 cups caffeinated tea or coffee toward goal

DAILY FOOD GROUP TRACKER

GROUP	FRUITS	VEGETABLES	GRAINS	PROTEIN	DAIRY	HEALTHY OILS & OTHER FATS	WATER & SUPER BEVERAGES
① Estimate Total							
② Estimate Total							
③ Estimate Total							
④ Estimate Total							
⑤ Estimate Total							
⑥ Estimate Total							
⑦ Estimate Total							

FOOD CHOICES

DAY ①

Breakfast: _____
Lunch: _____
Dinner: _____
Snacks: _____

PHYSICAL ACTIVITY steps/miles/minutes: _____

description: _____

SPIRITUAL ACTIVITY

description: _____

FOOD CHOICES   DAY ❷

Breakfast: _____
Lunch: _____
Dinner: _____
Snacks: _____

| **PHYSICAL ACTIVITY** steps/miles/minutes: _____ | **SPIRITUAL ACTIVITY** |
| description: _____ | description: _____ |

FOOD CHOICES   DAY ❸

Breakfast: _____
Lunch: _____
Dinner: _____
Snacks: _____

| **PHYSICAL ACTIVITY** steps/miles/minutes: _____ | **SPIRITUAL ACTIVITY** |
| description: _____ | description: _____ |

FOOD CHOICES   DAY ❹

Breakfast: _____
Lunch: _____
Dinner: _____
Snacks: _____

| **PHYSICAL ACTIVITY** steps/miles/minutes: _____ | **SPIRITUAL ACTIVITY** |
| description: _____ | description: _____ |

FOOD CHOICES   DAY ❺

Breakfast: _____
Lunch: _____
Dinner: _____
Snacks: _____

| **PHYSICAL ACTIVITY** steps/miles/minutes: _____ | **SPIRITUAL ACTIVITY** |
| description: _____ | description: _____ |

FOOD CHOICES   DAY ❻

Breakfast: _____
Lunch: _____
Dinner: _____
Snacks: _____

| **PHYSICAL ACTIVITY** steps/miles/minutes: _____ | **SPIRITUAL ACTIVITY** |
| description: _____ | description: _____ |

FOOD CHOICES   DAY ❼

Breakfast: _____
Lunch: _____
Dinner: _____
Snacks: _____

| **PHYSICAL ACTIVITY** steps/miles/minutes: _____ | **SPIRITUAL ACTIVITY** |
| description: _____ | description: _____ |

100-MILE CLUB

WALKING			
slowly, 2 mph	30 min =	156 cal =	1 mile
moderately, 3 mph	20 min =	156 cal =	1 mile
very briskly, 4 mph	15 min =	156 cal =	1 mile
speed walking	10 min =	156 cal =	1 mile
up stairs	13 min =	159 cal =	1 mile
RUNNING / JOGGING			
• • •	10 min =	156 cal =	1 mile
CYCLE OUTDOORS			
slowly, < 10 mph	20 min =	156 cal =	1 mile
light effort, 10-12 mph	12 min =	156 cal =	1 mile
moderate effort, 12-14 mph	10 min =	156 cal =	1 mile
vigorous effort, 14-16 mph	7.5 min =	156 cal =	1 mile
very fast, 16-19 mph	6.5 min =	152 cal =	1 mile
SPORTS ACTIVITIES			
playing tennis (singles)	10 min =	156 cal =	1 mile
swimming			
light to moderate effort	11 min =	152 cal =	1 mile
fast, vigorous effort	7.5 min =	156 cal =	1 mile
softball	15 min =	156 cal =	1 mile
golf	20 min =	156 cal =	1 mile
rollerblading	6.5 min =	152 cal =	1 mile
ice skating	11 min =	152 cal =	1 mile
jumping rope	7.5 min =	156 cal =	1 mile
basketball	12 min =	156 cal =	1 mile
soccer (casual)	15 min =	159 min =	1 mile
AROUND THE HOUSE			
mowing grass	22 min =	156 cal =	1 mile
mopping, sweeping, vacuuming	19.5 min =	155 cal =	1 mile
cooking	40 min =	160 cal =	1 mile
gardening	19 min =	156 cal =	1 mile
housework (general)	35 min =	156 cal =	1 mile

AROUND THE HOUSE			
ironing	45 min =	153 cal =	1 mile
raking leaves	25 min =	150 cal =	1 mile
washing car	23 min =	156 cal =	1 mile
washing dishes	45 min =	153 cal =	1 mile
AT THE GYM			
stair machine	8.5 min =	155 cal =	1 mile
stationary bike			
slowly, 10 mph	30 min =	156 cal =	1 mile
moderately, 10-13 mph	15 min =	156 cal =	1 mile
vigorously, 13-16 mph	7.5 min =	156 cal =	1 mile
briskly, 16-19 mph	6.5 min =	156 cal =	1 mile
elliptical trainer	12 min =	156 cal =	1 mile
weight machines (vigorously)	13 min =	152 cal =	1 mile
aerobics			
low impact	15 min =	156 cal =	1 mile
high impact	12 min =	156 cal =	1 mile
water	20 min =	156 cal =	1 mile
pilates	15 min =	156 cal =	1 mile
raquetball (casual)	15 min =	156 cal =	1 mile
stretching exercises	25 min =	150 cal =	1 mile
weight lifting (also works for weight machines used moderately or gently)	30 min =	156 cal =	1 mile
FAMILY LEISURE			
playing piano	37 min =	155 cal =	1 mile
jumping rope	10 min =	152 cal =	1 mile
skating (moderate)	20 min =	152 cal =	1 mile
swimming			
moderate	17 min =	156 cal =	1 mile
vigorous	10 min =	148 cal =	1 mile
table tennis	25 min =	150 cal =	1 mile
walk / run / play with kids	25 min =	150 cal =	1 mile

Let's Count Our Miles!

Color each circle to represent a mile you've completed.
Watch your progress to that 100 mile marker!

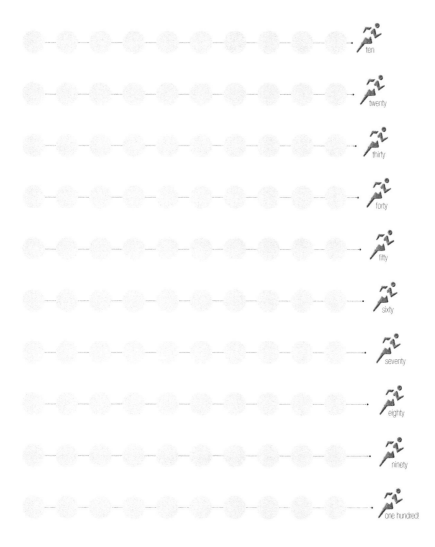

Made in United States
North Haven, CT
03 September 2024

56870606R00128